Arming the Immune System

The Incredible Power of Natural Immunity & the Fever Response

By Dr. Gurdev Parmar

To my family for their infinite love and support, allowing me to be brave. And to all the brave scientists and physicians who came before me, paving this road of knowledge.

Table of Contents

Introduction.......... 1

Chapter One: A Hot Topic.......... 13

Chapter Two: Getting Hotter.......... 27

Chapter Three: Fever for All!.......... 39

Chapter Four: Interrupting Fever.......... 51

Chapter Five: Suppression Means Staying Sick Longer.......... 71

Chapter Six: What's Really Going On?.......... 85

Chapter Seven: Fever Myths.......... 99

Chapter Eight: Benefitting from the Body's Natural Systems.......... 113

Chapter Nine: The Evolution of Fever Therapy into Modern Immunotherapy.......... 135

Chapter Ten: A Future with Fever.......... 155

Conclusion.......... 171

Acknowledgements.......... 179

References.......... 181

Introduction

It is the function of our intellect to realize the truth through untruths. Knowledge is nothing but the continually burning up of error to set free the light of the truth.

Rabindranath Tagore, poet and recipient of the 1913 Nobel Prize in Literature

As I sat in that lecture hall at Simon Fraser University, on the west coast of Canada, twenty-one years old and in my last year of my bachelor's degree in biological sciences, I knew I was about to have my mind blown. And I was ready. The class was called *Darwinian Medicine*, and I'd asked for special permission to attend. It was a master's course, and I was just an undergraduate, but I was fascinated by the subject and determined to learn. I was also a little star-struck by the professor.

Most people didn't know or care about Dr. Lawrence Dill, but to me, he was a celebrity. He was up there with the other giants, Drs. Ron Ydenberg, Louis Druehl, and Bernard Crespi. What—you haven't heard of them?

Maybe you're cooler than me. These guys were rock stars in the biology world back in the day. In my few years at SFU, they helped transform my understanding of our universe, world, species, health, disease, and more.

Now, I was about to hear directly from one of these rock stars of biology. Dr. Dill had graciously accepted me into his *Darwinian Medicine* class and was now pacing at the front of the room, looking every bit the superstar with his crumpled grey suit and fantastically bushy eyebrows. When he instructed us to open our textbooks, I had no idea that this book and course would be part of my transformation. It would help set the trajectory of my career and my research. It would lead to my writing this book— the one you are now holding in your hands— decades later.

The Body Does Its Job

The book was *Why We Get Sick: The New Science of Darwinian Medicine* by Randolph M. Nesse, MD and George C. Williams, PhD. The back cover said, "The next time you get sick, consider this before picking up the aspirin: your body may be doing exactly what it's supposed to." The authors were a medical doctor and an evolutionary biologist, and they discussed why things happen in the body from an *evolutionary* perspective.

They suggested that if you have a cough, there was a reason for it. Perhaps the body is prompting you to cough to help expel an infection in the lungs, and that stopping the cough may be counterproductive. They said if you have diarrhea because of an intestinal infection, this is the way the body rids that pathogen, and immediately stopping that diarrhea may not always be best. They said if you sprain your ankle and it gets big and fat, it might *not* be best to bring down the swelling, as the puffiness was preventing the ankle from moving which allowed it to stay in place and heal. They recommended that if you get a fever, you should not stuff yourself with fever-reducing medicines but instead let the fever ride, as it encouraged you to lie down at home, isolated and conserving energy to fight the fight. Ultimately, Drs. Nesse and Williams proposed that it is not always smart to blindly interfere with the body's natural processes. Instead, we should try better to understand and listen to these well-tuned systems that have evolved over hundreds of millions of years.

This text and course launched an obsession that had already been brewing in my young noggin' throughout my undergraduate degree. A captivation of the inextricable connection between humans, human health, and the natural world around us. After all, our bodies are complex ecosystems living within complex ecosystems. How can our bodies and their states of health be anything but completely dependent on the environment in which it lives? This connection has been unfolding for hundreds of millions of years and continues today. It's a story that explains why certain conditions or diseases exist and persist. Also, why our bodies do what they do.

Whether created in the image of god or by a magnanimous explosion, our bodies and the natural world around us are absolutely and positively beyond imagination or complete comprehension. Just incredible. Miraculous. Divine. This book and its subject matter applies to us all, regardless of backgrounds and belief systems.

More specifically relevant to this book, I was fascinated by the biological importance and significance of the many signs and symptoms we experience as humans. Each of them have good, solid, rational explanations for why they occur. I learned that it might not be best to always interfere with bodily functions that serve a purpose, including "symptoms" such as pain, inflammation, vomiting, diarrhea, and fever. Of all of these intelligent hard-wired programs we have in our bodies, the one that fascinated me the most, was the fever response. As I further explored my newly found obsession, I discovered exquisite research had been done across the animal kingdom, from insects and flies to humans of all ages, studying the incredibly complex and orchestrated mechanisms of our bodies in building a fever.[1]

Coalescing Ideas

Of course, as a premedical undergraduate student, I wasn't just taking one class with one textbook. My other studies included kinesiology, health sciences, philosophy of religion, and environmental toxicology. As I learned I constantly reconciled these new subjects with my ongoing interest in human health and the world around us. I was also fascinated with ancient teachings, human knowledge and wisdom through medical anthropology. I was starting to explore Ayurveda, Chinese medicine, botany and medicinal plant identification, and so on—practices that had developed over millennia. It is knowledge not to be lost. Yet, I have a naturally scientific mind. I like research papers. I need evidence.

Enter naturopathic medicine, a healthcare discipline that combines modern medical science with ancient medical wisdom. Naturopathic doctors (NDs) have foundations in anatomy, physiology, biochemistry, pathology, histology, and the like. Trained to perform complete physical examinations, lab tests, imaging tests, and able to prescribe pharmaceuticals and perform minor surgery. All of this built on the foundations of naturopathic philosophy rooted in traditional modalities including Ayurveda, Chinese medicine, herbal medicine, dietary and nutritional supplementation, lifestyle management, therapeutic fasting, hydrotherapy, and others.

With all these tools at hand, NDs can use standard diagnostic methods to form a diagnosis, then present evidence-guided and evidence-informed treatment options. Patients get the knowledge to make informed decisions. NDs guide them on who to talk to for conventional treatments and which natural and integrative options are available.

For all doctors, the first law, based on the Hippocratic oath, is: *First, do no harm*. That tells medical practitioners they shouldn't do anything more harmful than what is happening in someone's body. Treatments should not be more harmful than the illness. This idea underpins naturopathic medicine. The second, and just as vital tenant, is to cooperate with the body's own healing power—just as I had learned in the Darwinian Medicine course. When you understand what the body is trying to do, you can help it do its job. Sure, when things are broken, critical, or otherwise far beyond repair, modern medicine can take care of so much more today than ever before in all of history. But for most day-to-day chronic conditions and run-of-the-mill acute issues, listen, and help the body do its job, and stop stopping it all the time.

A Career in Cancer

Today I'm the co-founder and medical director of Integrated Health Clinic®. The Cancer Care Centre of our clinic specializes in naturopathic oncology—a distinct entity within the larger and broader discipline of integrative oncology. It's focused on evidence-based, whole-person care, and it uses all appropriate therapeutic approaches, healthcare professionals, and disciplines to achieve optimal health and healing.

We opened our clinic in 2000 and have treated tens of thousands of patients there. I'm licensed in BC, Canada, and Washington State, USA, and I've been a Fellow of the American Board of Naturopathic Oncology (FABNO) since 2007. Through this work with patients, other researchers, and educators, I am ever more interested in the benefits of *fever*. This might seem like a big leap from treating cancer, but from my perspective, it's actually integral to the subject.

The Path to Understanding Fever

Back when I was reading *Why We Get Sick*, I learned that fever is a natural, biological process found throughout the animal kingdom that has survived four hundred million years of evolution. I learned that this natural process is a beneficial treatment that the body creates for itself. As I became more interested in natural therapies, it made sense to look closer at what the natural fever process really does.

As I continued learning, talking to experts, and treating cancer patients and survivors, I further understand the incredible importance of fever in the immune system. Cancer, after all, affects the immune system. As do many other microscopic invaders, such as particulates, allergens, bacteria, viruses, and fungi. Our immune systems deal with these pathogens in an organized, efficient, and effective manner every day. Most of the time, our bodies are successful in shutting them down, preventing them from making us sick. However, once in a while, these tiny bugs or cancerous abnormal cells break through our bodies' first lines of defense, and infiltrate our systems. Just as it seems victory will be theirs, though, our bodies mount a massive response, overwhelming and destroying the invaders. This is the immune system at work, and fever is an essential element in its success.

The more I learned about the subject the more in awe I was of what the body can do. Fever is dismissed because it makes us feel bad, but it's an ancient mechanism for our defense, and we now have a massive amount of evidence that it is incredibly effective. It is powerful. It is safe. It is something every single person should know about. It's a tool we are all equipped with.

As time went on and my practice and experience continued to progress, I grew more and more intrigued by the world of immune-directed cancer therapies. I have now worked with forms of immunotherapy, a fancy term for treatments that directly affect the immune system—for almost a quarter century. I began clinical hyperthermia training in Europe in 2002. This was predominantly in Germany, but I learned from the world's foremost experts in hyperthermia from various countries representing Europe and Asia. We'll talk more about these treatments later in the book.

I conducted an eight-year retrospective observational study that looked at overall survival rates and quality of life for our clinic's patients treated for the most common stage four cancers, including breast, colorectal, lung, prostate, ovarian, and brain. The outcomes were published by Cambridge Scholars Publishing. I'm the lead author and editor-in-chief of a big book called *Textbook of Naturopathic Oncology: A Desktop Guide of Integrative Cancer Care*, which has a small section that dissects the many studies that demonstrate the benefits of fever, fever-inducing treatments, and all forms of immunotherapy currently in use in conventional oncology. That big ol' textbook was, however, for doctors. It used an obscene amount of nerdy words and impossibly boring tables and charts.

This book—the one you're holding in your hands—takes all the science, research, studies, and experience from around the world and throughout time and condenses it into something we can all understand and use. This book is a public service announcement. I wrote it for people who want to get sick less, get better faster, and live healthier lives. Yes, it's for doctors who want to treat patients better, but it's also for moms and dads caring for kids. It's for cancer survivors whose bodies have been ravaged. It's for people who can't afford to get ill. And it's for anyone who's ever been sick and didn't like it—which is all of us, right? Everyone on this planet will get some kind of sickness at some time, and the ancient mechanisms buried in our bodies will kick into action... if we let them.

An Exploration of Fever

In this book, you will learn that we *should* let our bodies' natural systems get to work because they are more effective at eliminating invaders than any military on earth. You'll discover that fever is an essential part of the immune system. We'll see how fever is found throughout the animal kingdom because that most powerful mechanism of the immune system is vital for survival. A fever is not just something to be endured; it's an ancient, beautiful, beneficial action integral to our bodies.

And this is true, even though fever feels awful. I mean, if you've ever had a fever, you know it feels terrible. It's noxious. I don't mean *nauseous* in that it will make you feel like vomiting (although it might). Fever feels *noxious*, as in, super uncomfortable. It's unpleasant. It feels bad. It might even be scary when you're hot and achy and clammy and sick. Especially given the fact that most people incorrectly believe fevers are uncontrolled and will cause seizures or brain damage. It's no wonder most people think we should suppress fevers as quickly as possible. I mean, who wants to feel like that? Who wants to risk brain stuff? Of course, people pop a couple of pills and whack a cold cloth on their head to reduce the fever fast.

Yet, in this book, we'll discover that except for very small and specific populations, there is *little to no evidence* in the scientific literature to support the idea that we should suppress fevers. Basically Zero. Zilch. There is certainly no irrefutable evidence in the history of humanity that says taking drugs to stop a fever is a good idea. In fact, there is a mountain of evidence that suppressing fevers makes us sicker for longer *and* makes sickness worse.

In these pages, we'll discuss the idea that taking medications to break a fever creates a short-term gain in exchange for long-term pain. We'll examine the science and myths around fever, discover what our bodies are trying to do when we're ill, and understand why so many people take medications to reduce fever, despite the lack of evidence that it does any good.

I'll share stories of bees who make an effort to fever together, lizards who lounge around trying to get a fever, kids who've had chickenpox longer than their peers because they took aspirin to stop their fever, and, incredibly, people whose cancer has completely disappeared after a fever.

It might sound too good to be true—and in some ways, it is. There are downsides to fever, too. Fever makes you feel like crap; we'll talk about why we should endure that. Yes, some kids do get seizures prior to their internal thermostats being fully developed. We will discuss this later. Some people with brain injuries may not be able to manage fevers. Same with certain elderly, frail, very ill, or emaciated patients. There are these exceptions, of course, but by and large, the downsides don't extend beyond just feeling crappy.

Being able to use fever to treat disease has also proven difficult, since fever biochemistry is complicated; it's horribly difficult for researchers and drug manufacturing companies to replicate what happens inside the human body. We'll discuss these challenges, how to overcome them, and my hypothesis of what will happen to the human race if we continue treating fever as something bad, and if we instead harness its power for our benefit. I think the science and studies—along with the miracle of the human body—will blow your mind as it has mine.

As I write, the world is in the midst of a pandemic, and it's vital we understand the immune response inherent in our bodies. I want us to have a healthier future. I want you to enjoy a healthier life. We start by honouring our bodies because they are incredibly intelligent, and they're working extremely hard for us. In the next chapter, we'll see how hard our bodies are working just to maintain our body temperature, and what happens when our internal thermostat intelligently and purposefully shifts to up the heat.

Chapter One: A Hot Topic

Give me the power to produce fever, and I will cure any disease.

Parmenides, Greek philosopher, circa 500 BC

Bees are amazing. Seriously. I got super into social insects, such as bees, wasps, and various types of ants, during my premedical studies. I know you think I'm crazy right now, but these little critters are ingenious. They have the best teamwork strategies on earth. Every bee works with its fellows to play its part in building the hive, growing the colony, and making that delicious honey. They even work together to fight infections.

There's a fungus called chalkbrood that kills off the larvae and mummifies them. It's caused by the spore-forming fungus *Ascosphaera apis*. You don't need to know the name, but I love Latin words, so get used to it. It makes it look like those baby bees have been covered in chalk and left to their death. The fungus doesn't usually kill older bees, but it can make them more susceptible to other diseases and prevents them from reproducing. When chalkbrood gets into a hive, it has the potential to be bad. Yet, it doesn't usually destroy colonies, as bees have a fantastic defense mechanism. The infection can't survive higher temperatures, so bees work together to create a kind of "social fever."[2] Inside the hive, they do this shaking thing. They flap their little wings, and their bodies jitter from side to side. I've seen videos. It's an incredible example of all for one and one for all.

As they vibrate, they get hot, and together they raise the hive's temperature by about 4 degrees Celsius. As we'll see later in this book, this has the same impact as the fevers you and I experience when we get sick. The fungus can't survive in the new temperature range. It dies, the larvae survive, and the hive lives on.[3] Bees are amazing.

So, what do a bunch of vibrating bees and *Ascosphaera apis* have to do with us? It turns out that from insects to fish, birds to lizards and snakes, and to every mammal, including humans, we all build fevers in response to infections. Unlike bees, humans do this without rubbing up against others—although that's always an option. But before we talk about how this deliberate temperature rise works, we first need to look at why temperature is relevant at all.

There's Effort Involved

Animal behaviour has a lot to do with temperature.[4] And when we consider this, we must remember that animals are either *endotherms*, with the ability to heat themselves, or *ectotherms*, without that trick. Ectotherms include fish, amphibians, reptiles, and invertebrates, and they're pretty limited on where they can live. They generally stay where there's plenty of sun, as they need it to heat their body and maintain their temperature. It's why you don't see many lizards in the arctic. Even fish, who sometimes live deep in the ocean, can only survive in the temperature zone they've evolved for and adapted to. A tropical *angel*fish can't hang out in glacial water; an *angler*fish—you know, the scary one from *Finding Nemo*—will die if the water gets much above freezing. Fish cannot control their temperature, so they must stay in relatively consistent environments.

That's not true for humans. We are endotherms. Between our bodies' biochemistry and our brains' evolved ingenuity, we can heat ourselves—and each other, if we're feeling bee-like.

Our endothermic nature means we experience physiological changes when we need to warm up or cool down. Our skin, hair, nerves, blood vessels, sweat glands, lungs, heart, and brain are all in on the act. We shiver to generate warmth in our muscles, and we sweat to cool our skin. Our blood vessels constrict to keep warm blood close to our vital organs when we're cold and dilate to do the opposite when hot. We shelter from the wind to warm up and pant like a dog when we're too warm. Through constant heat exchange with our environment via conduction, convection, radiation, and evaporation, our bodies are continuously making small adjustments to regulate our body temperature.

Our conscious behaviour affects our temperature management, too. The very early humans lived close to the equator. As humanity became more advanced, we adapted our behaviour to survive in almost any environment. We created shelter. We made big clothes for when it's cold and small clothes for when it's hot. We learned to heat food over the fire, drink tea to warm up, and sip iced tea to cool down. We engineered heating systems, saunas, air conditioners, and super soakers. We made humankind's greatest discovery: the recipe for ice cream.

Today, we have the technology to put babies immediately into incubators when they need to warm up. At the other end of life, when people are on their deathbeds, they have blankets pulled up and cozy socks on their feet. The youngest and oldest are most vulnerable to temperature changes, yet we still have ways to look after them.

From birth to death, consciously and subconsciously, we are all controlling temperature all the time. We constantly vary where we sleep, how we dress, what we eat and drink, and how we behave to accommodate temperature changes. And if you think about that, it's friggin' extraordinary. Wherever we have decided to live on earth, we can control our temperature there.

Under Control

And we *do* control our temperature. If you stick thermometers in people around the world, they all measure somewhere around 36 to 38 degrees Celsius.[5,6] All of them—unless they're sick, as we'll discuss. But assuming they're well, people in Kitimat, Canada, have the same body temperature as those in Koh Kho Khao, Thailand. We often take that for granted, but it tells us there is something incredibly valuable about that specific temperature range.

This temperature is where our biochemical reactions work as they should.[7] Our bodies manage an incredible number of processes every millisecond as they keep our organs working, our brains running, and our limbs moving. Every mechanism in our human bodies, every enzyme, every protein, every element inside you works best within this specific temperature range of 36 to 38 degrees Celsius. So, the body works hard to keep you there.

We see this in the numbers. Metabolic processes require about 1,800 calories a day. It takes about 60 percent of that to maintain our normal body temperature when in cold environments. That's a huge amount when you consider that the average adult in the Western world consumes about 2,000 to 2,500 calories a day. Temperature maintenance takes a large percentage of your daily energy. It's a tremendous amount of energy going to maintain body temperature. A 2021 paper called *Biochemistry, Heat and Calories* said, "Body temperature is tightly regulated by a process called thermoregulation, controlled by a master regulator, the hypothalamus that modulates the heat gain or loss by the body. Up to 60% of the heat generated during metabolic processes is used to maintain body temperature."[8]

Now, let's look at the American alligator. I know—you never expected to be compared to a reptile. While you're cranking out up to 1,800 calories on temperature control, this creature only expends about 60 calories a day on the same job.[9] You're using thirty times the amount of energy to achieve the same result. Alligators can get away without using much energy because they rely on the sun to keep it warm and water and shade to cool down. But where are these gators? Warm places close to the equator. Humans, as we know, are almost everywhere. Our bodies and behaviours have evolved to allow us to live in all climates, but we must compensate for the hot and cold by spending a ridiculous number of calories on maintaining temperature. For that process to have evolved, it must be bloody important. And it is.

I mean, just look at what happens when people are outside of this range. When someone gets really, really cold, they can't function. Their cellular mechanisms don't work. This is why it's so easy to die when you fall through ice into a freezing lake—your muscles can't work, and you can't swim.[10] When you get too hot, a similar response occurs, albeit in a different manner.[11] The body shuts down. It stops functioning. If allowed to get out of control, extreme temperature can lead to death. It's why you never leave a kid in a locked car in summer. Okay, there are lots of reasons not to do that, but possible overheating is one of them.

When your body is outside of this temperature range, it does everything it can, as fast as it can, to bring you back to normal. We do this in a preventative manner, too. I mean, instinct will stop you from just jumping into a bath. You dip your toe in first, right? If it's too hot or too cold, you yank your foot out of there pronto. When you first sit in your car, go to a hotel room, or into your office, you check the temperature. Temperature matters.

The Miracle of Measuring Temperature

How do we know we're all the same temperature? Well, we use thermometers. Today, these little gadgets are in almost every hospital, doctors' office, and home, but let's take a moment to consider the humble thermometer's importance and the utility of measuring temperature.

To understand temperature—and fever, as we will soon discuss—you must be able to measure it.

Doctors have been talking about and recording fever-like symptoms since ancient times. Parmenides gave the quote that opened this chapter sometime around 500 BC. Back then, doctors measured temperature by putting their hand on your forehead and asking if you felt hot. For thousands of years, people knew fevers occurred but couldn't measure them.

Then, in 1611, an Italian guy called Sanctorius wrote about his new invention: a thermoscope.[12] It was a massive contraption that used water, wine, or whatever liquid you had inside a glass tube, and the liquid moved when the temperature changed. Legend says it was inspired by Sanctorius's buddy, Galileo. Yeah, *that* Galileo. The exact details of the idea, the inventors' relationship, and possible other contributors aren't clear, but somehow, between brilliant minds, the earliest thermometer came into existence.

It couldn't report numbers as we know them—the Fahrenheit scale wasn't invented until a century later, and Celsius came after that—but it did verify the severity of a temperature change. Sanctorius used a mathematical equation that measured fluid displacement over time. He made the association that fast displacement meant the patient had a bad fever, and slower movement indicated they weren't so sick. Interestingly, Sanctorius also documented the temperatures of people who *didn't* feel ill. That's when he discovered we are all around the same temperature and started documenting normal and fever states.

A few decades after Sanctorius published details of his invention, Thomas Sydenham spoke up about fever. Sydenham wrote the textbook that defined medical practice in Britain for two centuries and is considered the "father of English medicine." Back in 1666, he said, "Fever is nature's engine which she brings into the field to remove her enemy."[13] He described fever like doctors before him had done for centuries: as more than just a symptom of illness. He said it was nature's way of annihilating illness.

The Battle of the Scales

The developments kept coming. At the end of that century, a guy called Carlo Rinaldini suggested that the melting point of ice and the boiling point of water should be the two fixed ends of a temperature scale.[14,15] That seems so obvious to us today, but it was a revolutionary proposition at the time.

Soon after, in 1724, Daniel Gabriel Fahrenheit came up with—you guessed it—the Fahrenheit scale for measuring temperature.[16,17] Being Canadian, I can't even describe it for you. He based it on some weird system that originally used 0, 32, and 90 degrees as points where water, ice, and salt changed states. I have no idea why he added salt to the mix, but his impossible math worked out, and we now had a consistent, reliable way to attribute numbers to temperature.

Anders Celsius wrote a paper in 1742 describing the Celsius scale, which used far more comprehensible math, with 0 and 100 as the two defining points.[18,19] Unsurprisingly, the world liked the easy math best, and Celsius was adopted almost everywhere except perhaps most notably the United States. So, by the late 1700s, there was a way for doctors to measure temperature. They could name and number it. What more did they need?

Identifying the Baddies

Nothing. Until a century later, when Louis Pasteur came along and shook things up. Pasteur is the French guy who's famous for developing vaccines, inventing the pasteurization process to stop bacteria from growing in milk and, importantly, wine, and doing a bunch of other impressive stuff that laid the foundations of modern medicine.

In 1861, Pasteur published his germ theory, which was a turning point in medical history.[20] He was the first guy to say that we get sick because of these tiny things called germs. Before that, the consensus was that sickness was caused by bad air, bad water, bad food, or imbalances of the body. People believed infections weren't passed from one person to another; they came from the air and environment around you, like the boogeyman sneaking up from the ground. At this time there was no such thing as antiseptic and people never washed their hands, let alone use sanitizer. So, Pasteur stood up and said something like, "Hey, bad germs are getting in us. That's what's making us sick. It's why we get fevers." And that led to an explosion of research on temperature and fever. We quickly understood that we were in an arms race: humanity versus germ. The war was on.

Soon after, it became standard for doctors to measure temperature as they tried to discern whether germs were winning the war on a patient. This happened in large part after a German doctor called Carl Reinhold August Wunderlich published a book called *Temperature in Diseases: A Manual of Medical Thermometry.* He had been obsessively measuring his patients' temperatures. This guy tested everybody, and he discovered that healthy people were always around 36 to 37 degrees Celsius—or, for our American friends, 96.8 to 98.6 Fahrenheit.

Wunderlich was super excited about this. Remember: this was before medical imaging like simple x-rays, blood tests, or urine tests were even a thing. Back then, all doctors had was a physical exam. Now, there was finally something measurable, objective, and reproducible. Plus, it was simple! You stuck a small stick in a patient's mouth and got a number that was either normal or not. And you know how much us doctors today like numbers. So, measuring temperature became standard medical practice around the world.

It seems it was all happening in Germany back then. Sixteen years later, another German guy, Carl von Liebermeister, made the distinction between hyperthermia and fever. For the rest of our discussion and the thesis of this book, this is key. He figured out there's a state where the body is hot *but doesn't want to be*, and there's a different state where the body is *actively trying to heat up*. The former is hyperthermia, and the latter is fever.

Almost a century later, E. S. Snell and E. Atkins[21] discovered there were actually four states of body temperature: normothermic, which just means normal temperature; hypothermic, where you're really cold; hyperthermic, where your body is hot but doesn't want to be; and fever, where your body is deliberately trying to be hot. They also proposed another idea that has stood the test of time since its inception in 1968: they suggested the body has a *set point*. Just like your thermostat at home is set to a specific temperature, the body has its own set point of 36 to 38 degrees Celsius. In normothermia, hypothermia, and hyperthermia, the set point remains the same, but environmental factors can change, making you feel just right, too cold, or too hot. In these states, no matter the environment, the body strives to maintain that normal temperature.

In the fever state though, the set point goes higher, and the body purposefully raises its temperature to reach the new set point. The body intentionally turns up its thermostat, then works extra hard to pump up the temperature and reach the new setting. Snell and

Atkins's set point idea has been consistently proven correct in subsequent studies that show that when humans are in a fever state, their bodies want to stay between 38.5 and 40.5 degrees Celsius, even when you try to cool them. We'll talk more about this fascinating set point change later.

Back to the Bees

With this information, the scientific community thoroughly explored and actively researched these four states of temperature. Physicians, biologists and physiologists began actively looking into these ideas. They conducted studies with humans and across the animal kingdom. This is how we know about the bees. Remember those incredible critters who vibrate together, creating social fever to save their babies?

But what exactly is this thing that has evolved in the last four hundred million years and that we see in bees and most other animals? Why do we all maintain a specific body temperature and set point? What is fever—beyond feeling hot and seeing a change in the thermometer? And how can we take advantage of the important ways in which fever is different from hyperthermia? Let's explore that next.

Chapter Two: Getting Hotter

Fever is a mighty engine which Nature brings into the world for the conquest of her enemies.

Thomas Sydenham, known as the father of English medicine, circa 1650

A long, long time ago, someone would get sick, and their loved ones would send for their village's medicine woman. The healer would arrive, ready to attend to her patient with preparations of herbs from ancient recipes and wisdom passed down through generations. Medicine Woman would feel her patient's forehead and, indeed, the patient was hot. "Are you sick, or have you spent too much time in the sun?" she would ask. You see, Medicine Woman had no way of knowing *why* a patient was overly hot. She couldn't distinguish between hyperthermia and fever.

As we learned in the last chapter, it wasn't until 1877 when our German friend, Liebermeister, discovered that these two states were distinct. In 1991, Matthew Kluger, author, physiologist, and one my favourite guys in the fever world, published an incredible paper called *Fever: Role of Pyrogens and Cryogens.*[22] We'll talk later about pyrogens and cryogens (these are the chemicals in our bodies that raise and lower our internal temperature), but Kluger succinctly summed up this essential finding in his paper. He said, "Leibermeister suggested that fever was not the result of an inability to regulate body temperature but rather the regulation of body temperature at a higher level." Fever is a regulated state, hyperthermia is not.

And, as we discussed, in 1968, Snell and Atkins defined *four* states of body temperature: normothermic, hypothermic, hyperthermic, and fever. (Get used to these words—you'll be hearing them a lot.) But why was it a big deal to distinguish between these states? Why did Medicine Woman want to know what made her patient hot? Because *the cause determines the treatment.* Understanding that your patient has overheated and is now hyperthermic, requiring immediate cooling, is critical. Perhaps more important is understanding when your patient is in a fever state and their body is deliberately trying to get rid of an underlying condition such as an infection. In that case, actively cooling them is not the best idea, and instead they require rest, isolation, and the chance to maintain their fever. So, let's look at the four states, their causes, and the treatments.

Just Normal

Normothermic means normal body temperature, which varies slightly from person to person and hour to hour, but it's around 36 to 38 degrees Celsius. It's kind of boring. Boring in a good way, sure, but it just looks... normal. Someone might get a little chilly if the wind picks up or want to take off their sweater when the heating kicks in, but they exchange heat with the environment in a steady state, never losing or gaining much before regulating back to the set point. Medicine Woman doesn't do anything for normothermic folks because there's nothing to fix. All animals called thermoregulators on earth maintain a body temperature of between 35 to 42 degrees Celsius.

Friggin' Freezing

Hypothermic, with an *o* in the middle, is when someone is colder than the normal set point of 36 to 38 degrees. Their body is trying to get back to normothermic, so it does a bunch of clever things to raise its temperature.

The person starts to shiver. That's their muscles contracting to generate heat. The blood vessels in the skin constrict. Blood vessels help us exchange heat with the air because, amongst many other things, blood is like the body's coolant. It's as if a car engine is pumping coolant around itself to control the transfer of heat.

When a patient is hypothermic, their blood vessels close down to prevent losing any more heat. They transmit as much heat as possible to the body's core, where essential stuff like the heart hangs out.

Without treatment, a hypothermic patient can lose consciousness. Their heart can fail, and their respiratory system craps out, and they can die. Death is bad, so Medicine Woman will load them up with the biggest, warmest blankets they can get find. They'll sit the patient by the fire, make them a hot tea, and wait for them to warm up.

Assuming the patient is still able to function, they might do this stuff for themselves. Hypothermia changes our conscious behaviour as well as bodily functions. It makes someone seek out warmth like a lizard looking for sun. It makes them ask Medicine Woman for a hot drink. It compels them to help themself if they can.

Super-Hot

You can picture hyperthermia, right? Imagine a person has been out in the sun too long, and they have heat stroke. Obviously, it's not a stroke, so I don't love that term, but you know what I mean. They've been out in the sun, they're dehydrated, their blood sugar's a bit low, maybe they also had a few too many margaritas making all that bad stuff hit overdrive, and we've got the perfect recipe for hyperthermia.

A lot happens here. Their temperature skyrockets and the body tries to let out this excess heat by opening the blood vessels wide. We call this *vasodilation.* It's the coolant kicking into overdrive. All those big, wide blood vessels make the skin appear pink, so on top of sunburn, they're flushed, too. They look like a lobster. Vasodilation takes blood away from the body's core and the head, so they feel like they're going to pass out. They want to throw up, and they're super weak. They're sweating buckets, their heart's racing, and every alarm bell in the body is screaming at them to cool down now.

The body is hot, but it desperately doesn't want to be, and this is a problem that needs correcting. If allowed to continue unchecked, hyperthermia can cause hypotension, shock, and even death if it puts pressure on preexisting conditions. Again, death is bad, so active cooling is a good idea. Medicine Woman is living in ancient times, so she doesn't have much to work with to help her hypothermic patient, but she'll want to whip out the cool cloths and go to town on tepid baths.

Feverish

In some ways, fever looks similar to hyperthermia. Our patient gets hot. They feel sick and weak and miserable. At one point, they sweat so much their skin looks like a slip 'n' slide. But there are some crucial differences. They don't start sweating *immediately.* In fact, at first, they feel cold and shivery.

Shivering is caused by acetylcholine (ACh) which causes muscles to burn brown fat and do this energy-expensive thing. Endotherms can do this, but *not* ectotherms. Thankfully, humans are the former remember? So, ACh gives our patient the ability to shiver to generate heat.

The weakness our patient feels is actually *exhaustion*. The body deliberately creates this sensation to encourage rest, which it desperately needs. For every one degree Celsius increase in body temperature, there is a 10 to 12.5 percent increase in basal metabolic rate (BMR). BMR measures the calories a body needs to function while at rest. While a fever creates a 4-degree rise in temperature, BMR can increase by 40 to 50 percent. That is a *lot*. In order for our patient to be able to fever well, they have to conserve their energy.

They want to bundle up. Remember: in a fever state, the body *purposefully* raises its set point, then makes itself hotter and hotter. The process causes behavioural changes, like bundling up in blankets, and physical changes like vasoconstriction at the periphery, which is the opposite of vasodilation. Blood vessels narrow to force blood to the all-important core of the body while simultaneously decreasing the loss of heat. The body does this until it reaches that new target temperature, and then our patient gets sweaty to stall the process and prevent overheating in the core.

In chapter six, we'll dive into the biochemistry involved in the fever process and explore these signs and symptoms further, but it's important to have an overview now. And it's vital to remember that unlike hyperthermia, hypothermia, and normothermia, fever is the *only state* in which the setpoint changes. Studies show fever consistently brings people to around 38.5 to 40.5 degrees Celsius. Even if Medicine Woman tries to cool her patient down, it won't work as the set point has increased. Interestingly all animal models from bees to alligators, birds, and fish – they all increase body temperature by an average of 2 to 4 degrees Celsius in a fever state, just like humans. There are differences in the normothermic temperatures of animals, but they all consistently increase by 2 to 4 degrees Celsius during a fever.

Determining the Difference

Medicine Woman is living a long, long time ago, and she doesn't know everything we do about fever. She can't determine the difference between fever and hyperthermia. If it's the latter, the patient will get hotter and hotter until they conk out. She can't just pop some fever-reducing medications in the patient's mouth, either; those haven't been invented yet. So, what does she do?

If she was smart, *really* smart, had the necessary tech, and way ahead of her time, she could figure out what Cooper discovered in 1964. After Leibermeister's and Snell and Atkins's publications, Cooper was one of the first to study this hyperthermia versus fever thing in humans.[23] He came up with an ingenious plan to understand what was going on.

Cooper took patients whose temperature was rising and immersed their arms in warm water. If you did this to a normothermic or hyperthermic person, their arms would turn red. Think of what happens when you get in a hot bath. Your skin goes pink as the blood vessels widen to let more blood—the body's coolant—circulate and release heat. This is vasodilation.

But in Cooper's study, the patients' skin *didn't* turn red. After being submerged in warm water, their arms still felt cool to the touch. When their bodies entered the fever state, they essentially changed their programming. Instead of responding normally, they now *prevented* vasodilation, so they didn't lose heat. Their blood vessels contracted away from the skin, bringing all that beautiful warm blood towards their body's core. Without as much blood near the surface, the skin felt cool. They were hot on the inside but cool to the touch. This was vasoconstriction.

We all know this from our own experience of fevers. Fevers have a heating stage, when the body is deliberately trying to get hot, and a maintenance stage, when the body's reached its new set point. In the heating stage, we shiver to generate more heat. We want to bundle up under blankets. The thermometer says we're hot, but we feel cold. Once the body's cranked its temperature above the new setpoint, it effectively goes into reverse to prevent the heat from escalating. That's when we start stripping off the blankets and sweating, which conducts heat away from the body and into the environment.

We don't react this way by happenstance. This is a sophisticated, deliberate, controlled heat management system. It's an orchestrated event. Even when we attempt to manipulate the process by artificially warming the body as Cooper did, the body won't let itself cool off. As long as we're not interfering with medications—as we'll discuss soon—the body very carefully controls its heating, cooling, and maintenance process. It's brilliant.

So, if Medicine Woman determines whether her patient has hyperthermia or fever, she can figure out the best way to treat them. Hyperthermic? Cool them down, stat. Don't let that thing get out of control. But if it's fever? The doctor can take a chill pill and let the patient be hot. The temperature won't escalate out of control. The patient's body is carefully managing the system in response to a specific trigger.

Triggering the Process

What triggers this temperature management system? We've touched on a few factors, and they're pretty common sense. Hypothermia happens when you fall through ice into a freezing lake or if you go outside in extreme cold without a winter coat. Hyperthermia is caused by heatstroke (not a real stroke). Fever can be caused by infections, malignancies, traumas, surgery, heat exhaustion, inflammatory conditions, autoimmune conditions, severe allergies, and unknown causes, too.

Most of all, fever is common because infections are common. Throughout our lives, we all get colds and cases of flu. We're exposed to any number of infections, so we get multiple fevers throughout our lives. This is true for everyone, everywhere, assuming their immune system and the fever-control area of their brain are healthy. No one is immune to all infections. There is no single human being who will go through life without ever getting a fever. People may choose to break that fever with medications, as we'll talk about soon, but not one of us will escape ever getting a fever in the first place.

Infections are most commonly caused by bacteria, viruses, fungi and parasites which can sneak into our bodies and interfere with our finely tuned systems. And these microbes are resilient little gremlins. They've been around longer than us, there are many, many more of them than humans, and they'll probably survive longer than us. They breed like rabbits—if rabbits took Viagra and gobbled up super-steroids. Some of them reproduce so fast they create thousands of generations in a single day. It's incredibly difficult for humans to keep up with them. Thankfully, we have a defense mechanism that has evolved over millions of years. The immune system operates twenty-four-seven, protecting us from the onslaught of invaders trying to get in. And fever is an essential part of that immune system.

Most bacteria and viruses die in the fever temperature range. Poliovirus, for example, can be killed at 40 degrees Celsius.[24] When its environment reaches that temperature, its reproduction rate reduces by 200 times. Fever is 38.5 to 40.5 degrees Celsius. Perfect. We'll talk later about the exact mechanisms that create fever and destroy bacteria and viruses, but fever kicks in to protect us from these little gremlins and keep us healthy.

Not only does the fever temperature kill off bacteria and viruses, but it triggers a host of other defensive processes. It increases the bactericidal action of neutrophils and other white blood cells that fight infections. That means your body kills bacteria faster. A fever temperature increases leukocyte or white blood cell production, function, mobility, and anti-microbial action, all of which helps these cells fight infection. And it increases acute phase proteins that create an inflammatory response, which is a complicated and well-orchestrated response to infections, amongst other things. The temperature increase also induces behavioural changes like aches and pains, fatigue, sleepiness, and anorexia (which, in this context, means no appetite) in order to conserve energy, forcing you to rest and isolate.

And it doesn't just work for us. The fever mechanism protects creatures across the animal kingdom. I'm talking hamsters, rats, guinea pigs, lizards, gators, crabs, scorpions, grasshoppers, lobsters, shrimp, beetles, leeches, snakes, snails, mice, monkeys, fish, ferrets, baboons, my beloved bees, and so many more. In the next chapter, we're getting into the animal world, and I promise, it'll be wild!

Chapter Three: Fever for All!

In all things of nature there is something of the marvelous.

Aristotle, philosopher, circa 1550

Did you hear the story of the peppered moths of London? It's a classic, taught in biology classes around the world. As it's been a few years since most of us were in school, and as Hollywood has yet to make it into a movie, let me tell you the tale of the peppered moths.

It's the early 1800s. We're in the city of Manchester, England. King George III sits on the throne. Manufacturing is the buzzword of the day. The Industrial Revolution is in full swing, thanks largely to the riches and resources taken from India—my family's homeland—and other imperialized countries. (Not that I have a chip on my shoulder) Farming families flock to Manchester to work the "well-paid" city jobs, and there are plenty of them—well, jobs, at least, if not well-paying ones. Factories are popping up in all the industrial areas. Fueled by burning coal, their chimney stacks pump plumes of black smoke into the sky. The heavy, dirty air fills factory workers' lungs, and the soot turns streets, horse carts, and even tree trunks black. And that is a problem for the peppered moth.

The peppered moth, you see, is a creamy white colour, with little black specks peppered across its wings. The pattern camouflages it beautifully against pale tree bark. But as trees in industrial areas turn black from pollution, the white moths can now be spotted a mile away. That's handy for the birds circling the skies, searching for tasty moths for dinner.

While no one was monitoring the survival of moths in the early 1800s, someone *was* watching them a few decades later. R.S. Edleston was an English naturalist who, like me, thought insects were pretty cool. In fact, he went several steps further and took his butterfly net out on insect hunts. In 1848, he wrote in his diary, "Today I caught an almost totally black form of *Biston betularia* near the centre of Manchester."[25] Now, I said you'd be getting some good ol' Latin names. *Biston betularia* means—you guessed it—*peppered moth.* I don't know why he was searching for insects in the heart of a booming city. Surely the countryside would've given him more to look at. But I'm glad he was there because this was the first time a black peppered moth had ever been recorded. They were supposed to be white. All of them! But no, Mr. Edleston caught a black one. And this guy knew his critters—it was definitely the peppered moth.

By 1895, Edleston's finding had become common. In industrial areas, up to 98 percent of peppered moths were this new beautiful and stunning black variety. Scientists had a great time trying to figure out the mystery of the colour-changing moths. Were they white but covered in soot? Were they eating that toxic crap and turning black? Was something messed-up happening to the larvae?

No. Eventually, a bunch of scientists came to the same conclusion. The colour change was due to a typical and expected genetic mutation which provided a survival benefit.[26] As with all living organisms, genetic mutations are a common occurrence during the process of cell division. Sometimes mutations can be a bad thing, but sometimes mutations are just what the doctor ordered. Where the trees were covered in soot, white moths were easily eaten by birds. Some of the peppered moths underwent a DNA mutation which changed their colour to black. These rare black moths survived those devilish birds, able to live another day and reproduce, creating more black moth babies. The original cream-coloured peppered moths became yummy treats for birds, and over a few decades, the black moths took over the species.

Evolving to Survive

This was evolution by natural selection in action. An environmental change happened: the trees turned black, and a creature became adapted to survive better in the new environment. In 1978, the American geneticist

Sewall Wright called it "the clearest case in which a conspicuous evolutionary process has actually been observed."[27] And that's why the story of the moths is so famous. Most evolutionary adaptations can't be observed within one human lifetime. They occur over much longer periods, measured in multiple generations.

Evolution describes how everything on earth changes over that time, and those changes occur through the process of natural selection, which conserves elements that allow us to survive. For example, if someone is bigger, stronger, faster, smarter, has better eyesight, hearing, hunting ability, physical attractiveness, or a colour that hides them from preying birds, these attributes are generally passed on to their kids. There's complexity in how our kids turn out, but natural selection tries to preserve the elements that make them more likely to survive.

We see this everywhere. In a pride of lions, the strong ones live, the runts don't make it, and the species self-selects to become stronger. Those funny-looking frigate birds have big, red necks, and the bigger the bulge, the sexier they look to the chicks. The process ends up favouring big necks, and the trait continues. Birds of paradise don't have fancy necks, but they dance like idiots to attract a mate, and wouldn't you know it, the species has produced the world's finest movers and groovers. Check them out on YouTube if you don't believe me.

But animals don't just need to reproduce. They need to live. They have to survive infections, and that's where the evolution of fever comes in. The fever process has survived four hundred million years of natural selection. Just look around during flu season, and you'll see that fever is thriving. It is a staple of our biology because *it is essential to our survival.* Just think: if it weren't essential, it would not occur. As we already discussed, it takes a great deal of our available energy just to maintain our normothermic body temperature. For a fever to increase our energy demand by 20 to 50 percent, it must be critically important. If it didn't provide us with a survival benefit, it would not be found in *all humans and all animals* that have evolved over hundreds of millions of years.

All Humans and All Animals

Yes, you read that right. All humans and all animals that have been tested by science. Even fleas get fevers, just like you. We know this because there has been an absolute ton of research into animals and the fever response.[28] Those creatures I listed at the end of the last chapter—hamsters, rats, guinea pigs, lizards, gators, crabs, scorpions, grasshoppers, lobsters, shrimp, beetles, leeches, snakes, snails, mice, monkeys, fish, ferrets, baboons, and my beloved bees—are just a few examples of animals that have been injected with bacteria, viruses, or lipopolysaccharide, and developed a fever.

Lipopolysaccharide is a ridiculously long word, so we call it LPS. LPS is a chemical found in the cell walls of what we call *gram-negative bacteria*. It is a major component of the bacterial outer membrane. It makes up about 80 percent of the outer membrane of E. coli and Salmonella, for example. It is also the most abundant antigen (the thing our immune systems build an immune response against), and it plays a very important role in the host-pathogen (antibody-antigen) response.

It took scientists a really long time to figure out what happens when bacteria enter the body, but they did it in part by looking at specific bacteria known to cause profound fevers. *Streptococcus* is one of them. That gives you strep throat and a wicked fever along with it. When scientists analyzed this bacteria they found LPS in the cell walls. They extracted this chemical, inserted it into a bunch of animals, and the poor creatures got fevers. They've now repeated these tests with more animals and fever-inducing elements than I can count. Every animal model tested develops a 2- to 4-degree Celsius rise in their body temperature if injected with bacteria, viruses, fungi, and cancer cells.

Dr. Philip A. Mackowiak is an emeritus professor of medicine. In 2000, he wrote an amazing paper[29] in which he described how this 2- to 4-degree fever response has been documented in vertebrates (animals with spines), arthropods (without spines), and annelids (like worms). If we follow the progress of evolution, we see species branching off into their own lines of development at various stages in history. If the fever response is shared between these three phyla of the kingdom Animalia—these three major branches of the evolutionary tree—we have to go all the way back to before they branched off to find a time when they were one organism developing this one characteristic. To find that common branch of evolution, we have to go back *four hundred million years*. That's when these types of animals split off into their own evolutionary lines, taking the fever process along with them.

Humans have spines, so we fall into the vertebrate category. And like other vertebrates, when we get sick, our bodies raise our temperature by 2 to 4 degrees. For such a well-controlled mechanism, this is a massive change, and it takes an extraordinary amount of energy to make it happen. Again, when we're talking a 10 to 12.5 percent increase for every degree raised. So, for a 4-degree increase in body temperature, the caloric demand increases 40 to 50 percent. You'll remember from chapter one that in a normothermic state, you spend about 1,800 calories a day to maintain your temperature in a cold environment. Now, increase that by 40 to 50 percent for a fever temperature increase, and you're spending calories faster than you can take them in. In fact, during a fever, the body induces a lack of appetite to conserve energy for the immune system's response as it puts a ton of energy into purposefully increasing your temperature.

An Incredible, Orchestrated Response

So, every human and basically every animal fevers, and it takes a huge amount of energy. Wouldn't it be ridiculous for all animals to spend that much energy on something that *wasn't* completely necessary? Of course. Atkins (that researcher from the last chapter) and another of her colleagues, Phyllis Bodel, said, "It is difficult to believe that this universal response [fever] of warm-blooded animals would have survived if it did not, indeed, serve some useful purpose in combating disease."[30] There is copious research that demonstrates the benefits of fever, and we'll discuss all that later in this book, but common sense alone says that if fever weren't required for our survival, the fever process would have died off a long time ago. And it didn't. It has survived hundreds of millions of years of evolutionary development. If it were just in humans, that would be one thing, but the fever response plays out across the animal kingdom.

Now, perhaps you don't put much stock in evolution. I would imagine that no matter your belief system, you have an immense respect for the way our bodies have been tooled. Whether you have a religious affiliation and believe strongly in creation or take a more naturalist approach to your worldview, I think we can all agree that our bodies are amazing. We are all equipped with this beautiful system that, amongst a million other things, maintains our core temperature on a moment-by-moment basis and adapts our temperature when we're sick. However we came to achieve such an incredibly orchestrated response, this is truly an amazing defense mechanism unlike anything we humans could ever hope to artificially produce.

Fever Equals Survival

Even in simple organisms, we cannot perfectly reproduce the fever process. Take sponges, for example—you know, like you find on a coral reef. They look like plants, but these plain, old, squishy sponges are animals *that fever.* They don't even have any organs, let alone limbs or a brain, but somehow, they've figured this fever survival stuff out. And fossils show they've been around for about six hundred million years, so I think they're doing okay for themselves.

Here's the fascinating thing, though (as if sponges aren't already interesting enough): If you were to infect a sponge with LPS and its temperature rises, and then give it a fever-reducing medicine like aspirin, the fever would go down… and the sponge would die. The bacteria is allowed to take hold, the infection runs rampant, and the sponge actually dies. Goodbye, sponge.

We see this response across the animal kingdom. Take lizards, for example. Now, remember they are ectotherms, which make great temperature study subjects since controlling their body temperatures is much easier than in endotherms. In ectotherms, by controlling the heating and cooling sources, one can control their temperature.

In one study,[31] researchers took a lizard tank and used artificial lights to replicate the sun's heat. On one side of the tank, they set the temperature to 50 degrees Celsius, and on the other, 30 degrees. They plopped in a few healthy desert iguanas and watched the reptiles waddle back and forth between the heat zones to maintain their normal lizard body temperature of around 36 degrees. If they got too cool, they shuffled over to the hot zone. Once they warmed up, they headed back to the cool area without any human provocation.

When the researchers injected these desert iguanas with the bacteria *Aeromonas hydrophila*, which makes these iguanas sick, those scaly little guys hit up the hot side of the tank and stayed there. They didn't budge until their body temperature hit 38 to 40 degrees, or a fever state. That's what we expect by now, right? They want a high body heat to kill off the invading bacteria and to activate the immune system, but they can't control their own temperature, so they use the environment to force themselves into a fever state. Next, these researchers gave the iguanas the antipyretic (anti-fever) drug acetylsalicylic acid (ASA). They found when they prevented the lizards from getting hotter than their usual 36 degrees, the little guys died. Only those iguanas who were able to fever despite the ASA survived. Those that weren't able to fever died.

A similar study was conducted on New Zealand White Rabbits.[32] (Sorry, I know they are cute, and science can be mean, but stick with me here, please) Researchers infected the rabbits with *Pasteurella multicide*, then gave half of them intravenous saline and the other half intravenous sodium ASA. Not surprisingly, 100 percent of the rabbits given sodium ASA died of their infection, compared to 29 percent of the control group who were given saline and were able to mount a fever.

Okay, one more example to drive this point home. In a study on ferrets infected with a recombinant influenza A virus,[33] researchers measured the viral levels (or *viral shedding*) in the nasal washes of the ferrets. Again, half of the ferrets were allowed to fever. The other half were given sodium ASA and were shaved to bring down their fever. Yes, they shaved the poor creatures to remove their furry warm coats! They found a significantly higher level of viral shedding and a longer duration of sickness in the ferrets actively treated with fever-reducing medicine and a good, sharp shave. Wait for it, as similar studies have been done on humans with various infections, and we'll get to that later on in this book.

In the world of medicine, we refer to allowing a fever to happen without interruption as "letting it ride." When animals are *not* allowed to let their fever ride, they succumb to the invading infection and die. Mackowiak summed it up when he wrote that, "There is considerable evidence that fever is an important defense mechanism that contributes to the host's ability to resist infection."[34]

There is evidence of this across the animal kingdom, and yet... you might be thinking that we *humans* don't die when we don't let it ride. If you get a fever and pop an ASA to bring your temperature down, you don't conk out like a lizard. And clearly, we are more complex than your average sea sponge or flea. So... what does happen? What do we need to know about fever in humans?

The experience is so commonplace that many people assume they understand everything about it. They never think to question what their well-meaning parents taught them, or what they read on the side of a pill bottle or saw on a TV advert. But in truth, much of the information proliferated about fevers is rooted in myths and misconceptions that are repeated and reinforced over time. Until the late 1800s, fever was widely considered a healthy sign during disease. This view has changed with fever-lowering drugs now the knee-jerk reaction worldwide. We have more scientific evidence than ever about what actually happens when people fever—and when they interrupt this natural process with common, easily-accessed medications. So, let's talk about these medications and what really happens when we interrupt fever.

Chapter Four: Interrupting Fever

> *Two critical assumptions are made when prescribing antipyretic therapy. One is that fever is, at least in part, noxious, and the other is that suppression of fever will reduce, if not eliminate, the noxious effects of fever. At present, neither assumption has been validated experimentally.*
>
> **Philip Mackowiak, Physiological Rationale for Suppression of Fever, 2000**

One evening, my wife and I were curled up on the couch watching the latest episode of one of our favourite shows when a commercial came on for a brand of acetaminophen for infants. It showed all these cute little babies with rosy cheeks smiling dolefully after their loving parents soothed them with a dose of medicine. The message seemed to be this: you can make your child feel immediately better just by giving them this product. And they'll also be endlessly adorable and happy. And that's the lesson we're all told, right? If your kid has a fever, give them some meds, they'll feel instantly better, be super happy, and life will be full of rainbows and unicorns. Who wouldn't want that? My wife and I have four children, and we sure want them to feel good. It's heartbreaking when they're sick. We want to do all we can for their comfort.

That commercial and millions of others like it promise that if you take a medication, it will almost immediately take away every symptom of sickness. Fever, chills, aches, pains, and everything else that feels bad will disappear. And, for the most part, it's true. These medications are in a class called non-steroidal anti-inflammatory drugs (NSAIDs, which you can pronounce in your head as *en-said*. It's less hassle than listing each letter every time). Amongst others, they include acetaminophen, paracetamol, ibuprofen, naproxen, diclofenac, and ASA. You might be more familiar with brands than these generic names, but I'm going to avoid brand names out of fear of being quietly murdered by some suits. As with most households around the world, you probably have a few of these pills kicking about your bathroom cabinet, so check the labels to see which medication is in each brand-named product. But exactly what you have might depend, in part, on your medical history and where you live.

What's In A Name?

Living in Canada, acetaminophen is commonly used for anything from headaches and fevers to hangovers and hockey injuries, and virtually all other minor aches and pains. However, I've spent a lot of time traveling around this incredible planet, including many trips with my family to Thailand, where we built and volunteered at a small clinic after that devastating Boxing Day 2004 tsunami. Much of our clinic's medications for each of the trips were supplied by an awesome NGO called Health Partners International, from Quebec, Canada. They provided our small, upstart H.E.L.P. Foundation with wonderfully thought-out boxes, each packed with enough Canadian drugs to treat hundreds of patients for many of the most commonly seen issues. Not only did we treat the local Thai, but we were on an island with many Scandinavian, German, and Australian tourists who also attended the clinic—all of whom were completely confused whenever I prescribed acetaminophen. "What the hell is this?" they'd ask. Apparently, there is a great worldwide divide over which drugs are most popular where. In each of these countries, as with many others, paracetamol is the standard equivalent.

Although the various NSAIDs work in slightly different ways, they are all antipyretics (meaning they reduce fever) and analgesics (they reduce pain). The mechanisms of action of each drug in this class are slightly different, nuanced, and, yes, complicated, like everything in the body. We will be talking at length about how this all goes down in chapter six, where we'll get right into the biochemical science behind how NSAIDS reduce fever and pain. But for now, let me start with the two main mechanisms of NSAIDS. First, these medications inhibit enzymes inside you called cyclooxygenases (COX enzymes), which decreases an ever-so-important prostaglandin (or fatty acid) called prostaglandin E2 (PGE2).

Let's start with the COX group of enzymes. There are several variations of this enzyme, imaginatively called COX-1, COX-2, and so on. One of the primary functions of these enzymes is to convert something called arachidonic acid (the stuff that makes your muscles sore after a hard workout) into a fatty acid called prostaglandin H2 (PGH2). PGH2 is what then gets converted by the body into other molecules, including PGE2. So, long story shorter, COX enzymes make PGE2.

Why is PGE2 so important? Because PGE2 is given most of the credit for shooting up into the temperature control centre of the hypothalamus, called the pre-optic area of the hypothalamus (POAH),[35,36] and getting it to increase the thermal set-point of the body. As we all know by now, this is the critical step in creating a fever, and is what separates fever from hyperthermia. Amazingly, the POAH is just a tiny part of that already only pea-sized hypothalamus. Yet despite its miniscule size, it has the massive responsibility of adjusting the thermal set point and creating a true fever response. Just wow.

As I mentioned earlier, NSAIDs interfere with the COX enzymes' ability to produce PGE2. Without that PGE2, the hypothalamus lowers the fever thermal set point back to normal, which brings your temperature down, taking away all the aches and pains with it, and voila. You feel better.

Ibuprofen, diclofenac, ASA, and other drugs in this class are effective for reducing the symptoms of fever, yes, but they are also very useful for improving symptoms more in the body's periphery—you know, all the dangly bits. If you have arthritis in your fingers or a severe tennis elbow from too much... well, tennis (no, I don't know anything about that), these drugs work well for reducing inflammation. You may know that ASA is also used to "thin the blood," which can be helpful for people who've had a stroke or a heart attack, or otherwise want to prevent blood clots. It actually prevents platelets from getting sticky in the blood, but most people understand that it has the effect of thinning the blood, so there you go.

The other NSAID option is acetaminophen. Or, if you're on the other side of the great, worldwide divide, paracetamol. These two drugs behave differently than the other NSAIDS. Their mechanisms of action works less on reducing COX enzymes directly and more on the central nervous system. The effect is that they're typically a bit less effective for aches and pains in the dangly bits, but more effective for central pain, like headaches.

However, from a fever perspective and for the purposes of our discussion, we don't really need to differentiate between the nuances of the various types of NSAIDs. Yes, they operate in different ways, but their approach to interrupting fever is essentially the same, and, perhaps more importantly, they give us the same outcome: reducing fever symptoms. If you've got a fever and pop any of these pills, your temperature will come down, and your aches and pains will ease.

The Somewhat Embarrassing Truth

Although we will dive into the complex biochemistry of the fever process in chapter six, I can't actually share much more about the mechanisms of action of NSAIDs. I have already described much of what we understand about COX enzymes and PGE2, the role these play in fever, and how NSAIDs interact with the process. These are the bulk of relevant details we actually know. The truth is that we don't yet completely understand how each of the NSAIDs work. We do understand that there is more going on here. What's that? You're saying the body and its functions are complicated, perhaps more complicated than we currently understand? No, don't be silly.

In one study,[37] patients with a fever were given NSAIDs to suppress their fever. Then, they were given a dose of PGE2. The hypothesis was that if they replaced the PGE2, the patients' bodies would be able to continue to fever, despite the NSAID. But it didn't work. Even when researchers replaced PGE2, the NSAIDs somehow overcame it and *still* suppressed the patients' fevers. This illustrates that there are multiple mechanisms at play in increasing the set point. We know PGE2 is an important factor, and that NSAIDs inhibit its production. But we don't understand exactly what else is going on. And that's just crazy, considering some of these drugs have been around for more than one hundred years, and are amongst the most widely used medications in the world year after year. It is a bit shocking that with all the medical understanding at our fingertips today, we still know so little about some of the most widely used drugs on earth. NSAIDs are available over the counter. They're in everybody's hands. Anyone can buy them, and most people do. Including doctors. It just goes to show the incredible complexity of the human body.

If you want to know more about NSAIDs and fever, I recommend going through the paper that describes this study. (The reference is included at the end of this book.) Long story short, PGE2 is not the only endogenous pyrogen. We know that tumour necrosis factor, IL-1, IL-2, IL-6, and others are all endogenous pyrogens capable of creating fever (hold on to your seats, you will learn about each of these soon). These all remain in play.

The Advent of Aspirin

The advent of the drug found in the popular product Aspirin came in 1897. But the journey to this incredible medicine started a handful of millennia earlier. People have been using willow bark to treat fevers and other ailments all the way back to the ancient Sumerians and Egyptians.[38] Willow bark is one of thousands of natural plant medicines that has long been used by healthcare providers and knowledgeable people around the world. Prior to the 1900's, natural medicines were all we had. Humans intelligently and methodically figured out which kinds of plants, fungi, animal products, and factors from our natural environment provided some medical benefit for particular ailments. That knowledge was passed from generation to generation. Even today, many pharmaceutical drugs owe at least part of their discovery or production to a naturally occurring, non-patentable product.

With scientific progression, we figured out there was this chemical in the bark of the willow tree called salicylic acid. As the field of chemistry became more robust, Felix Hoffmann, a German chemist working for the company Bayer, was able to make salicyclic acid less bad tasting and easier on the stomach, by making acetylsalicylic acid (ASA), and gave us the earliest form of Aspirin. At the time, Bayer was largely a chemical company occupied with the extraction of dyes from coal tar, but it had started a small pharmaceutical arm. As the story goes, Hoffman's father was dealing with rheumatism for which he took the long-used, bad tasting, and hard on the stomach medicine called sodium salicylate. To help his father, Hoffman wanted to find a better tasting drug that was not so hard on the stomach, and through his employment at Bayer, he was able to develop just that. He called it ASA.

That was the all-important 1897 development, and doctors loved it. Of course, they did. Imagine it: A person comes in with inflammation, you give them one of these drugs, and their inflammation goes down. Perfect. And it worked for all sorts of inflammation and pain. Toothache, headache, sore throat, swollen anything... You got an ache? We got your medicine, baby.

From 1899 to 1956, ASA had its heyday. It enjoyed fifty years of virtually no competition in the pharmaceutical world. Then, in 1956, acetaminophen and paracetamol came along and stole a huge part of the market share. In 1962, ibuprofen was developed and took its share of the market, too.

There are a number of drugs in common use today that are extracted from plants, and those plants have been used for thousands of years without anyone knowing exactly which chemical constituents provide the benefit. Being most familiar with the drugs used in oncology,

I can think of several examples of commonly used chemotherapy drugs that come from plant medicines. The chemo drugs called *microtubule inhibitors* include the Vinka alkaloids from the Madagascar Periwinkle flower (*Canthanthus roseus*), Paclitaxel from the Pacific Yew tree (*Taxus spp.),* Docetaxel from the European Yew tree (*Taxus spp.),* and Maytansine found in Kadcyla, which is derived from the Maytenus flowering plant (*Maytenus ovatus*). There are other types of chemo drugs called *topoisomerase inhibitors*, which include the drugs irinotecan and topotecan. They're both known as Camptothecins, and they both come from the Happy Tree (*Camptotheca*). The drugs etoposide and teniposide are extracted from the May Apple tree (*Podophyllum*). That's a lot of today's most commonly used chemotherapy drugs that come from plants.

Over millennia, our ancestors somehow figured out the almost unknowable. Their incredible and sublime work led medicine to the drugs which today continue to be an important part of the armamentarium in use against most cancers. All those years ago, people had no idea about the stuff in these plants and what it exactly did inside of us. They just figured out that this thing worked. Eventually, pharmaceutical companies started producing drugs, and they didn't always know why those worked, either—just that they did. Often the drugs come first, and the full understanding follows. There's something incredibly intelligent about the human ability to determine what works even without the benefit of scientific evidence. This type of knowledge is passed down through generations. "If you drink water steeped with this plant, your cough will get better. I don't know why, but it works." What a credit to humanity that we had reached these conclusions without the benefits of biochemical labs.

Doctors, Patients, and the NSAID Love Affair

Doctors want to make their patients feel better. And NSAIDs are a wonderful tool for making aches, pains, and fevers disappear. Of course, doctors recommend them. If a patient comes in feeling like a dog's breakfast, just terrible, and you give them a drug that makes them better in twenty minutes, you're a hero. Then the patient says, "Wow, thanks, Doc. I feel so much better. I'm so happy you gave me that stuff. You're awesome." The patient leaves feeling better, and the doctor feels like a superhero for destroying those ugly symptoms. We all want to reduce our patient's suffering.

It's not just us doctors that love that these drugs work—everybody loves that NSAIDS work *so darn well*. People want to avoid pain; NSAIDs reduce pain. They work fast; there are very few things that provide such immediate relief. Think of other common ailments like heartburn, diarrhea, or constipation. You can take stuff for those symptoms, but they rarely work so fast and so consistently effectively. NSAIDs, though? Give them twenty minutes to kick in, and you're good to go. And that applies to basically everybody that takes them, all the time.

They are generally safe and well tolerated, too. Well, ASA can be very bad for infants. It can cause Reye's syndrome, which is rare but potentially fatal for little ones. In large doses acetaminophen is not good for the liver. But otherwise, NSAIDs are relatively safe medications. They're cheap and readily available. You can just grab them off the shelf in most countries or get them over the counter without a prescription. Yes, almost everyone loves NSAIDs, and it's no wonder they've become a standard of care for many issues, and some of the most widely used medications in the world.

Mackowiak, that researcher dude I mentioned earlier who wrote about the evolution of fever in vertebrates, arthropods, and annelids, wrote many papers on this subject. In one, he said, "A little less than a century later [after the development of ASA], the marketplace is replete with drugs capable of suppressing fever. Their widespread application by primary care physicians, emergency department nurses, pharmacists, parents, and other caregivers has been at least in part motivated by a general suspicion that fever is inherently noxious. This suspicion is reflected in the results of surveys reporting that approximately 40 percent of parents and other caregivers regard temperatures encountered during fever as harmful."[39]

There is no evidence to support the idea that fever temperatures are harmful. Literally none. And I don't mean *literally* like when you say your head will literally explode if you have to hear me say this again. I mean absolutely, completely, literally-by-the-dictionary-definition, not a single piece of evidence for this. In fact, there's evidence *against* it, which I'll show you in the next chapter. In the same paper that Mackowiak gave us that quote, he reports that an estimated 70 percent of nurses and 30 percent of physicians regularly use antipyretic (fever-reducing) drugs. With all these medical professionals and regular folks using NSAIDs, it's no wonder they have been a multi-billion dollar a year business worldwide. That's a heck of a lot of NSAID use.

Safe, But Not Completely

These drugs are not without disadvantages—and some potentially major ones, too. According to StatPearls Publishing, "Acetaminophen toxicity is the second most common cause of liver transplantation worldwide and the most common cause of liver transplantation in the US. It is responsible for 56,000 emergency department visits, 2,600 hospitalizations, and 500 deaths per year in the United States. Fifty percent of these are unintentional overdoses. More than 60 million Americans consume acetaminophen on a weekly basis, and many are unaware that it is contained in combined products."[40]

This happens because at doses greater than four thousand milligrams a day, acetaminophen is potentially toxic to the liver. Another concern is how many people use these drugs for their hangover headaches. After a heavy night on the booze, their livers are already toxic from trying to process so much alcohol. Then, you throw in the added stress of too much acetaminophen, and sometimes the liver can't handle it.

NSAIDs can also be really hard on the stomach. They can eventually cause ulcers, which are holes in the stomach lining. They hurt—a lot—especially when you eat or drink. Which, you know, you need to do to survive. Ulcers can bleed, too. The blood goes into your digestive system and can turn your stool black and tarry. You can even start vomiting blood. You can lose so much blood you collapse and wind up in hospital in an emergency situation. Yes, these rare side effects happen with chronic NSAID use. They take time to develop and are largely avoided by managing the much earlier and minor symptoms of gastritis (inflammation of the stomach), but this does happen to some. In fact, in the long term, NSAIDs can be hard on the kidneys and heart as well. Yes, they're generally relatively safe, but we shouldn't fool ourselves into thinking that they're totally benign. They are not. Even in generally healthy people who don't have hangovers and take nice, responsible, low doses, there are very real issues.

The Problem with Masking Symptoms

In March 2020, when the world was wrapping its head around the novel SARS-CoV-2 (COVID-19) pandemic, the US Food and Drug Administration (FDA) spoke about this. It released a statement offering advice for people concerned about how NSAIDs may worsen infection from the COVID-19 virus. There was speculation in the media and amongst the public that NSAIDs might worsen lung problems and other symptoms of COVID-19. This concern followed a March 11, 2020 letter in *The Lancet* medical journal that hypothesized that NSAIDs could aggravate COVID-19 symptoms. With this concern out there, many people who wanted to take NSAIDs to reduce their COVID-induced symptoms, including fever, did not.

There has since been subsequent further discussion that, "NSAID use is not associated with higher mortality or increased severity of COVID-19."[41,42] In the medical community, studies need to be supported by other, better controlled and larger trials with greater participant numbers to further support a hypothesis before being accepted. As I write, we don't yet have definitive evidence from such trials. Yet one thing *is* clear to me: NSAID use masks COVID-19 symptoms, which increases the chance of transmission. If you feel fine because you popped NSAIDS, you're more likely to go out and about, accidently spreading your germs to all you encounter.

The FDA spoke about another problem in the same sort of vain. They said, "All prescription NSAID labels warn that the pharmacologic activity of NSAIDs in reducing inflammation and possibly fever may diminish the utility of diagnostic signs in detecting infections." In other words, there is an inherent risk in taking an NSAID that a doctor won't be able to tell what symptoms you actually are having, and therefore might not diagnose and treat you appropriately.

The Therapeutics Initiative is a Canadian organization that provides up-to-date, independent, evidence-based, and practical information on healthcare interventions. They said the same thing when everyone was asking for advice on treating COVID-19 symptoms. In this quote, I've skipped some of the less relevant details for the sake of length, but you can see the full statement online.[43]

"Many people are asking doctors for information about whether it is safe to use NSAID drugs now. ... Feeling an increase in your body temperature can tell you if you are sick. And, fever is an important vital sign which can alert doctors and nurses about your clinical condition. However, it is not usually medically necessary to suppress fever. ... Relieving fever and treating pain are comfort measures that can help people stay active and/or maintain good eating and sleeping patterns but are NOT needed to shorten the duration of illness."

The statement continues, "Use NSAIDs only if the advantages for pain truly outweigh the potential disadvantages. Remember that it is rarely necessary to lower your temperature. Fever is one of the key vital signs that allow nurses and doctors to recognize whether a sick patient is improving or worsening. If you are sick and need to seek advice or treatment, measure your temperature (if you have a thermometer), and your heart rate, and be prepared to report them accurately."

People get so mad when a doctor misdiagnoses them, and rightly so. It's a big deal. But what if our patients are masking their symptoms and making it almost impossible to make accurate assessments and ultimate diagnosis? Many people do this without even realizing it. They're just trying to get through the day without feeling so crappy, but they're inadvertently creating problems by masking their symptoms.

This isn't a new problem. In 2015, a study was published which looked at severe *Group A Streptococcus* bacterial infections. That's strep throat, and if you've ever had it, you know it causes a wicked fever. Researchers discovered that patients treated with NSAIDs ended up with much more severe infections than those who did not take them, and instead let their fevers ride. Doctors were better able to assess the severity of the infection in those who did not take NSAIDs. It proved difficult for doctors to understand the degree of infection when symptoms were suppressed. They just couldn't tell what was going on.

Typically, with a Group A Streptococcus infection, doctors will put people on antibiotics. If it's a severe infection, they'll deliver them intravenously. You can imagine what happens, right? If a person is given an NSAID, their fever drops, and they don't feel that bad. They tell the doctor they're fine. But inside, they're brewing this nasty infection. The doctor's usual diagnosis tool of assessing the degree of fever is gone, so they have to trust the patient when they say they're okay.

Let's play worst case scenario again. What can happen when that patient doesn't get adequately treated? They could get sepsis, an infection in the blood. And then you have a hospitalization, a whole bunch of complications, all which could easily have been avoided with a simple and appropriate antibiotic treatment, if only the doctors had known they needed to administer it. So, yeah, it can be crucial to be able to see the signs and symptoms of illness. When a doctor or patient can't tell what's really going on, they're at a huge—and potentially very dangerous—disadvantage.

Perhaps an even bigger issue that comes to my mind is the larger public health concerns of sick people harbouring viral infections but masking their symptoms with NSAIDs. These drugs are so effective at taking away most symptoms of the infection that they allow infected folks to go about their daily lives—which includes going to work, school, and everywhere else in their communities, innocently transmitting the virus wherever they go. This is what I was talking about above with COVID-19. What would happen if people stopped using NSAIDs every time they were sick? Would they do a better job of isolating? Would transmission slow down? I suspect yes to both. As far as I know, this hasn't been studied (possibly because it would be difficult or impossible to design a study looking at this potential harm), but common sense tells me that we should take note. As you know by now, the symptoms the body creates during a fever basically force us to rest and stay home, isolated from the rest of humanity. Our bodies want us to do the best thing for our own bodies *and* for our loved ones and community.

It Gets Worse

It's not just that infections get worse when we can't properly identify them and that we're likely to transmit those infections to more people. There's a growing mountain of data that suggests the act of reducing a fever can directly cause an infection to run for longer. We'll dive into those studies in the next chapter because they are fascinating. And not just for science geeks like me. I think they will prove very informative for anyone—okay, basically everyone—who's grown up being told to just take a few pills, and you'll feel fine.

Because here's what we're *not* told in all those cute baby commercials, by doctors who genuinely want you to feel better, and by caregivers who want to help you get on with your busy day: *Not a single NSAID will cure what caused your fever in the first place.* If you're sick and take one of these drugs, you'll start feeling more like a regular human being, sure, but your body will still be under attack. The bug that penetrated your defenses is still there. It's hidden. We can't see the signs and symptoms, but it's still attacking.

Maybe that doesn't seem like a big deal. "Who cares that I'm still sick if I can't feel it?" That's a fair question, and here's the answer: *you* should care. You really should. Me, too. All of us. Because suppressing a fever is a short-term gain for a long-term pain. That is my contention. Suppressing fevers means staying sick for longer. Not convinced? That's okay! It may sound like kind of a wacky idea if you've never heard it before. In the next chapter, we'll dig into the evidence.

Chapter Five: Suppression Means Staying Sick Longer

> *[T]here is considerable evidence that fever is an important defense mechanism that contributes to the host's ability to resist infection.*
>
> **Philip Mackowiak, Physiological Rationale for Suppression of Fever, 2000**

One would think that with the universal and routine use of NSAIDs to treat fever, there must be an Everest-sized mountain of high-quality, peer-reviewed evidence to suggest this was a good idea. Turns out, that is not the case. There is, however, evidence to the contrary: That when you suppress the symptoms of a fever you actually stay sick longer—and that the sickness can be worse than it otherwise would have been. Now, when I say *evidence*, I don't mean one oddball study with arguable results, but I also don't mean an Everest-sized mountain either. For reasons we'll explore in chapter eight, this topic has not been investigated with much interest in the medical community. Given the fact we all get sick, and that most of us routinely use NSAIDs, it warrants much more attention. Nonetheless, the weight of the existing evidence points to suppression of fever as a culprit in staying sicker for longer. That's huge, right?

Okay, off the box of soap I come. Let's get right into what we know, to give you some juicy conversation starters for your next party. Imagine yourself with a cold beer in hand and a group of fascinated friends around you, hanging on your every word as you say, "Did you know that suppressing fever, which is actually really good for you, keeps you more sick for longer...?"

Sick for Longer

Did you know that kids who get chickenpox will likely be sick for longer if you give them acetaminophen? True story. This was the finding of a study published in the *Journal of Pediatrics*, aptly and succinctly called *Acetaminophen: More Harm Than Good for Chickenpox?*[44]

This was one of those randomized, double-blind, placebo-controlled trials, which is awesome. These trials are the gold standard in medical research. In these studies, half the participants get the tested drug or protocol or whatever, and the other half get a placebo. It's totally random who is assigned to which group. Researchers can't pick and choose who gets the real treatment or the placebo, and neither them nor patient knows who's getting what. This prevents subconscious (or deliberate) biases. In medicine today, only randomized, double-blinded, and placebo-controlled trials are widely accepted as reliable evidence of treatment effect.

In this 1989 trial on children with chicken pox, researchers gave thirty-seven children acetaminophen and thirty-one children placebo for six days. They measured itching, appetite, activity, overall condition, time to last vesicle formation (blisters forming), time to total scabbing (blisters crust over), and time to total healing of the exanthem (full-body rash). Their conclusion? I'll let them tell you in their own words: "These results provide evidence that acetaminophen does not alleviate symptoms in children with varicella [a virus that causes chickenpox] and may prolong illness." Nonetheless, most children around the world with varicella continue to use acetaminophen and other NSAIDs to treat their chicken pox.

And it's not just chickenpox that shows this result. There was a fascinating study published in *The Journal of Infectious Diseases* by Stanley et al.[45] in which they took a real, hard look at snot. These dedicated, hard-working researchers poked away at test tubes of nasty nasal mucus samples from people with rhinovirus, which is the main culprit for the common cold. Researchers measured how much of the virus was in the mucus. They call it measuring *viral shedding*—patients literally shed the virus out of their bodies via mucus. [Quick aside, this is a primary defensive mechanism provided by mucus. The mucus traps the virus, bacteria, or other offender, allowing it to be sneezed, blown, coughed, vomited or pooped out of us.] Back to this rhinovirus study: As long as the snot still contained virus, the patient was deemed still sick. When the mucus tested clear, the virus was gone. This is an objective and more reliable way of assessing for active infection and sickness duration, than simply monitoring symptoms. So, what happened when these researchers dug into the snot? They found people treated with ASA shed the virus for longer. As in, *they were sick for longer.*

Then, Stanley and his colleagues did this study again. Presumably this wasn't because they particularly loved handling this particular bodily fluid, but because they wanted to corroborate their results. And they did. They got the same results the second time around. Here's their summary:

> *In two double-blind trials, volunteers challenged with rhinovirus were treated with aspirin or placebo. Aspirin treatment did not alter the rates of infection or illness but was associated with a moderate reduction in the frequency or severity of some symptoms.*
>
> *The overall benefit in rhinovirus infection was not statistically significant. Aspirin treatment appeared to cause a highly significant increase in the rate of virus shedding in treated subjects. The increase in virus shedding must be considered an adverse event that could influence the course of the disease in the individual and increase the likelihood of the spread of the infection to contacts.*

Another rhinovirus study is surely what you want right now, so here is one more for you, this time published by Graham et al.[46] It was also a double-blind, placebo-controlled trial, but this time the researchers wanted to see if these same results occurred with other types of NSAIDs, using ASA, acetaminophen, and ibuprofen. Guess what? They too came up with the same results.

They took sixty healthy volunteers and exposed them to rhinovirus type 2, which seems a little sadistic, but the participants were taking one for the team. Thanks, guys. Fifty-six of them got sick, and researchers gave them one of these three medications or a placebo, then watched how long the virus was active. The team reported, "Use of aspirin and acetaminophen was associated with suppression of serum neutralizing antibody response ... and increased nasal symptoms and signs." They went on, "There were no significant differences in viral shedding among the four groups, but a trend toward longer duration of virus shedding was observed in the aspirin and acetaminophen groups." So, none of the NSAIDs made people better faster, and two out of three actually had the opposite effect, making people sick for longer than those who were allowed to let their fever ride by only getting a placebo.

For more proof of concept, let's look at some of the evidence in support of the idea that patients unable to mount a fever, and who have a lower peak temperature while sick, have worse outcomes. Bryant et al. did a retrospective analysis of 218 patients with gram-negative bacteremia.[47] They found that a low or normal body temperature during bacteremia (infection with bacteria) was associated with increased mortality. What does that mean in normal language? People were more likely to die when they were unable to mount a fever. Mackowiak and his team found the same thing when they analyzed 184 cases of polymicrobial sepsis (mixed bacterial blood infection).[48] Taking the concept one step further, Weinstein et al. found a positive correlation between a temperature of greater than 38 degrees Celsius and survival.[49] Supporting the idea that the hotter people are able to get when sick, the more likely they are to live.

The Unfinished Study

A particularly noteworthy randomized controlled trial published in 2005 by Carl Schulman et al. in the journal *Surgical Infections* evaluated the impact of antipyretic therapy on critically ill patients.[50] A total of 82 patients were randomly assigned to an aggressive treatment group (44 patients) or a permissive group (38 patients). When people in the aggressive group got a fever of 38.5 degrees Celsius, they received 650 milligrams of acetaminophen every six hours. If their temperature reached 39.5 degrees, they also got a cooling blanket in addition. The permissive group, however, were left alone to let their fever ride. Only if they hit 40 degrees did the researchers intervene and give them acetaminophen and cooling blankets, but otherwise, the researchers just observed that group.

What were the results? We don't know completely as they had to terminate the study early. They had to. At the interim analysis, seven participants had died in the aggressive treatment group, and only one person had died in the permissive group. The study had to be stopped early due to "issues of waiver of consent and the mandate for minimal risk."

Now, I want to be clear: I'm not saying the study caused or contributed to these deaths. The human body is complicated, and the study participants were already sick. It's noteworthy and beyond chance that there was such a significant difference in mortality rates between the two groups. And remember, patients were randomly assigned. It's not like all the sickest people were placed in the aggressive treatment group. Granted, this is a relatively small sample size and the study was never finalized, so it doesn't provide firm conclusions, but it is interesting and further proof of concept, further supporting the other studies with similar findings.

Other NSAIDs

"What about ibuprofen?" I hear you cry! Well, in the previously mentioned Graham et al. rhinovirus study, ibuprofen didn't help people get better faster, but also didn't prolong illness. It was the acetaminophen and ASA groups that made people sicker for longer.

Well, we now get a closer look at ibuprofen in a 1997 trial titled *The Effects of Ibuprofen on the Physiology and Survival of Patients with Sepsis: The Ibuprofen in Sepsis Study Group* published in the *New England Journal of Medicine*. In this industry, getting into that journal is a pretty big deal. It's like our equivalent of winning the Pulitzer Prize or something.

This study took place in hospital locations across the United States from 1989 to 1995. It was randomized, double-blind, placebo-controlled trial. Again, all good stuff. It studied participants with sepsis, or infection of the blood. Because the bacteria are circulating in the blood, they get everywhere, and sepsis is bad news. These patients are *sick*.

Over the six years, half the patients in this study got ibuprofen and half received placebo. Researchers measured body temperature, heart rate, oxygen consumption, urine tests, and a bunch of other data. After thirty days—you guessed it—there was no difference in survival rates between the two treatment groups. The ibuprofen didn't help anyone live longer.

It did some other interesting things, though. It lowered patients' temperatures. Not a good thing in my opinion. We expect that though—it means it's effective in reducing fever. It also decreased heart rate, reduced the amount of inflammatory elements excreted in urine, and decreased oxygen consumption. These three factors are interesting because they are all measurements of certain aspects of a healthy immune system response. Instead of being allowed to get on with business, and kicking in the high heat, a higher heart rate and higher oxygen consumption, with the requisite inflammation; all these factors were suppressed, making it harder for them to help the body heal. Plus, the ibuprofen did nothing to prevent shock or respiratory distress—which are the big things that kill people with sepsis. It lowered the immune response and didn't prevent death. That's kind of kick in the teeth, right?

The Big Picture

For those of you that would like more information on this stuff, there's a cool paper called *Fever: Suppress It or Let It Ride* by Juliet. J Ray and Carl I. Shulman, published in *The Journal of Thoracic Disease* in 2015.[51] It summarizes a bunch of this data in an easy-to-read format, and it's available for free online. The link is in the references at the back of this book. I recommend checking it out for a quick overview of the subject. Plus, it's less than three pages long. You can't say I give you too much homework.

However, for a broader overview we will look at a systematic review. These types of publications are really important. They're where a group of researchers look at the available data on a research question and review it for common trends, weird discrepancies, or some semblance of consensus. They allow the reader to see the big picture summary of the experts after their review of all the individual studies, all in one place.

Jonathan Dallimore et al. published a systematic review and meta-analysis in 2018 called *Effect of Active Temperature Management on Mortality in Intensive Care Unit Patients.*[52] In normal language, that means it asked if treating a fever with NSAIDs helps sick people live longer. In short, the answer was no. When these researchers reviewed the available research on this question, they concluded the individual studies were not anomalies. The results were consistent. Fever management simply did not help people live longer. The only exception was in people with acute brain pathology, which we'll talk about in chapter seven. Aside from that tiny population, fever management had no bearing on who died and who survived, nor how long a patient stayed in hospital. The only thing shown was that NSAIDs successfully lowered body temperature and provided some symptomatic relief. They did what they promised, but that didn't significantly help anyone.

There's No Blame Here

I want to make it clear that no one is no finger-wagging here. There's no blame towards anyone for using NSAIDs for themselves, their kids, or their patients. For a hundred years or so, we've all just been doing what we've been told or taught is best. "If you're sick, take these pills." Every one of us has done this, and it's completely understandable. My parents treated some of my fevers with NSAIDs, and knowing the data in this chapter, I don't begrudge them for it. They just wanted to make their little children feel better. They were loving parents trying to do their best for their children. My wife and I have also administered NSAIDS to our four boys for various reasons through life. Can you relate?

When we know better, though, we can do better. Now, we know that fever management is not necessarily always the best idea. This book is a *public service announcement* to help more and more people discover these facts for themselves, possibly changing their patterns in how they manage fevers in the future. By sharing these studies and finding out more, by taking the time to read books like this one, we can help each other leave behind old misbeliefs and become comfortable with the natural, beneficial mechanism of fever.

We don't need to keep blindly repeating what we were taught by parents or professors who repeated whatever they were taught, who learned from the generation before them. Let's instead start a conversation around these studies, so we can learn from the science.

One Overwhelming Fact

Physicians are really good at dissecting studies, and it's true that you'll always find people who can form an argument for or against anything they see. Those discussions are important as they help us assess which research is reliable. I hope that if you're interested, you'll also dissect the studies listed at the end of this book for yourself. Nothing beats seeing black-and-white results first-hand.

But while we're analyzing all this research, let's keep in mind one overwhelming fact: Fever has survived four hundred million years of evolution across the animal kingdom. Fever exists because it's essential for survival. Its continued ability to thrive no matter how our bodies or environments change, is kind of hard to argue against. As much as we have clinical evidence from all these studies, the real proof is in the pudding, as they say.

So, we know that using NSAIDs to lower fever doesn't make any difference to any important outcomes, and that infections continue for longer when we use NSAIDs. As Mackowiak succinctly put it, "Clinical data supporting an adaptive role for fever, although sparse, include evidence of both the beneficial effects of fever and the adverse effects of antipyretics on the outcome of infection."[53]

He wrote that more than twenty years ago, when the data was sparse. The research in this space over the last few decades has continued to grow, though. Although I'm calling for more attention for this subject, many people have recognized this as an area worthy of investigation, and we now have much more research confirming what was clear to Mackowiak even then. When you use these medications, you're getting a double-whammy: you don't get better faster *and* you're sick for longer. This is good to know—really good, because who wants to stay sick longer than necessary?

This isn't to say NSAIDs don't work. They do exactly what they're supposed to. They're extremely effective at lowering body temperature during a fever and reducing aches and pains. The point is that reducing fever and pain doesn't help where it matters. It doesn't make you better faster. It doesn't get you discharged from hospital and back home sooner. And it doesn't make you more likely to survive a serious infection.

All we can say is it makes people feel better, which sounds, on the surface, like a good thing. But—and here's the real kicker—I believe it is lowering your chances of dealing with severe infections in the future. This is my hypothesis, which I'll share in detail later in this book. To understand why this idea is serious, though, we first need to talk about what really happens during fever from a biochemical perspective. When you understand the nitty-gritty of the fever process, you'll see why so many myths exist around the subject, how we can actually benefit from fevers, and why the future looks pretty bad if we continue to suppress fevers for the sake of feeling a bit less achy in the moment.

Chapter Six: What's Really Going On?

Fever is perhaps the most ancient and widely known hallmark of disease. For much of history the word 'fever' has been used almost synonymously with disease itself as various epidemics have ravaged the civilizations of East and West alike.

Elisha Atkins and Phyllis Bodel,
Fever, 1972

In an orchestra, the conductor stands front and centre, surrounded by musicians who watch her every move as they simultaneously read music and play beautiful symphonies. I don't know exactly how they can do all that at once or how they understand what the conductor is doing. To me, it just looks like she's flapping a stick around. But apparently every move she makes, every twitch of the wrist or pinch of fingers has an intended response from the entire orchestra. The musicians all understand what they should do according to these movements. In an orchestra, every little thing means a lot. It's all essential to the symphony. Fever is a beautiful biochemical orchestra. It's one part of the body sending small but significant signals to a multitude of other areas, which all instantly know what's required of them. They work together, each playing their part in creating the symphony of a fever response.

I've held off sharing the details of this biochemical orchestra until now because, frankly, it's pretty geeky and will be tough slogging. We're about to go deep into the science. I'm going to tell you about the cells and chemicals involved, how they work, and what we know about the fever process. I'll also share the mysteries that research hasn't yet figured out. If you want to check out the research papers that support this, I recommend starting with *Pathogenesis of Fever*,[54] which is probably the most succinct and up-to-date review of the biochemistry of fever.

In this chapter, though, we're going deep so that by the time we're done, you will truly understand that fever is a deliberate mechanism integral to the immune response—and one that we should *cherish*. When I think about this stuff, I feel incredible reverence for the human body. It's amazing and harmonious and complicated and beautiful. I hope this will show you why the body—*your* body—is so wonderful, and why you should trust in its wisdom.

Bad Guys Attack

The biochemical mechanism of fever is really a great story—an incredibly complex organized response that includes various parts of the body, cell types, and chemicals. The fever story starts once upon a time when a person—you, let's say—gets an infection. We can all get fevers from infections, malignancies, traumas, surgery, heat exhaustion, inflammatory conditions, autoimmune conditions, severe allergies, or the catch-all "unknown causes." But for the purposes of our story, we need some bad guys, and bacteria are a great choice because they're so commonplace. Those little gremlins get everywhere, and they're well-studied by science. Also, I'm writing during the COVID-19 pandemic, and I think we've all had enough of viruses for a while. So, enter the bacteria.

You'll see this in the scientific literature. The vast majority of such research is done using bacteria. These bad guys are easy to work with. Viruses go into cells and mess up all sorts of stuff we don't fully understand yet, making the outcomes difficult to unravel. Bacteria are more straightforward, though. You can take them, dead or alive, inject them into a subject, and they will cause a fever. You can even just extract lipopolysaccharide (LPS), the chemical in certain bacteria's cell walls, and that alone will trigger a fever. This all makes bacteria easy to work with for fever research.

And for the sake of our story, let's get more specific, and say the bad guys are *gram-negative bacteria*. This is the type of bacteria that contain LPS, whereas gram-*positive* bacteria don't have LPS, being made up of different bits and pieces. In addition to having that fever friendly LPS, the gram-negative bacteria have been used most in research, so we understand them quite well.

Okay, so we've got the good guy (you) and the baddie (gram-negative bacteria), who are carrying a dynamite bag full of LPS. One day you're out doing something brave and exciting. Maybe you're surfing at Stinky's beach in Punta de Mita, Mexico, escaping sharks and the giant diving pelicans (no, of course this is completely fictional). Imagine you make an impressive surf of a monster wave, riding it like a champ with the entire beach on pause watching your epic ride. Then you hop off your board, walk out to your adoring fans, and slice your foot on a barnacle-infested rock. Naturally, you don't let on, continuing to strut with board held high and easy. But that barnacle has sliced your foot good.

Ah-ha! Gram-negative bacteria now have a way into your body. They enter through the wound. Once inside, they encounter a bunch of your internal, brave soldiers called white blood cells (leukocytes), which include lymphocytes, neutrophils, and macrophages. These leukocytes are floating around your bloodstream and hanging out in tissue. They act like little Pac-Man guys, eating up bacteria and other bad stuff that enter the body. Chomp, chomp, chomp. Perhaps the most well-studied type of leukocyte is the macrophage.

How do your white blood cells know which things or cells are foreign invaders? The plot thickens. All our cells are surrounded by membranes that have a very specific pattern like a fingerprint. They are unique to the cells of our own bodies. White blood cells have what are called *pattern recognition receptors*. These receptors can distinguish between the very specific pattern of our "self" cells and the "non-self" patterns.

So, the baddies get in. Our Pac-Man cells identify them as "non-self" stuff, and start eating them up. As they eat them, they gather their information—their unique pattern—to share with the rest of the immune system. And as they're munching away, the Pac-Man guys release cytokines into your blood. Cytokines are the chemical messengers used by cells to communicate with other cells. With cytokines, cells can send information to various and distant parts of the body. That's how the hip bone can talk to the thigh bone and whatever else that song says. Cytokines basically send messages telling the cells in the rest of the body, "Hey, we got a problem here!"

Action Stations!

The cytokines involved in fever are called endogenous pyrogens (EP). *Endogenous* means from within, and *pyrogen* is a substance that makes the body produce fever. You can remember EPs by thinking of them as little pyromaniacs, setting you on fire from the inside. A guy called Paul Beeson, who was a preeminent academic physician both in the US and the UK, discovered and named EP in 1948. He figured there was something in the body causing a fever biochemically, and he and a bunch of other researchers around this time were able to isolate this thing, but they didn't really know what it was. They just knew that if they took EPs and put them in your hypothalamus, you got an instant fever. Interestingly, they also found that if you injected EPs into the neck, the fever was a little bit delayed, and if you put them into the feet, the fever was even more delayed. They thought whatever these EPs are, they work in the brain. Ingenious start.

Then, in 1972, researchers Igal Gery and Byron Waksman further investigated EP and finally named it interleukin-1 (IL-1). Why did they name the previously called EP "*inter-leukin*-1?" Since this is a cytokine that allows *leuk*ocytes to communicate with each other, they *inter*act between *leuk*ocytes, and we get *interleukins*. Hey, who said scientists were creative? There are now lots of interleukins that have been identified—over thirty of them last I checked. However, we still give IL-1 a ton of the credit for mounting a fever response. We now also know that there are several other families of EPs including tumour necrosis factor (TNF) and prostaglandins like PGE2.

You keeping up with all these names? If not, don't worry. The goal here is to give you an idea of the system. The science-y words are just gravy. Anyway, these five EP messengers (IL-1, IL-2, IL-6, TNF, and PGE2) trigger a whole bunch of things to ramp up. For example, the body starts producing more neutrophils, another type of Pac-Man-like white blood cell, increasing their munching action. They also increase the production and munching activity of natural killer cells, lymphocytes, and dendritic cells. Dendritic cells take the information ("fingerprints") gathered by all these Pac-Man-like cells from the invading cells and share it with the real killers, the memory cells that kill and never forget who they don't like. They're trained killers with specific targets that remain their targets.

These five EPs (IL-1, IL-2, IL-6, TNF, and PGE2) also produce heat shock proteins that "prime" the cytotoxic T Lymphocytes. What does that mean? The EPs unfold proteins on the invader's cell membranes, changing what they look like and allowing trained cancer-killing cells to recognize these heat shock proteins as non-self. Once they find the non-self proteins, they arrest them and then present them to the rest of the adaptive immune system, so they can't be forgotten. Basically, there's a ton of action going on with all the cells of the immune system: the innate (Pac-Man) cells, the bridging (dendritic) cells, and the adaptive (cytotoxic T lymphocytes) memory cells.

While these immune cells are doing their thing, the five chemical messenger EPs are going straight to the brain. They head for that little hypothalamus, which, as we've talked about, is a pea-sized part of the brain tucked behind the forebrain. And we can get even more specific. They go to the pre-optic area of the hypothalamus (POAH), which controls body temperature. (But as we know, the process can't take place 100 percent in the POAH, as there have been studies in which the POAH is surgically removed and there is still a fever response to intravenous infusions of EPs similar to controls.[55] It seems the brainstem and other parts of the brain step in and do the job we typically credit the POAH for doing. Nonetheless, while there is a POAH in the brain, there is no doubt that a majority of EP action lies right there.

Now, once the EP messengers get in there, they need to firmly latch on to transmit their message. That's what receptors are for. EPs are cytokines, and all cytokines act as "keys" that float around until they find a lock on another cell that they can fit into. When they do that, they open a door into the cell to perform certain functions. Cool, right?

Back to our five EPs of interest. Once our Pac-Man-like cells find that gram-negative bacteria, they release these EPs into the blood, which float right up to the brain, work their way into the POAH, and attach to receptors (locks). When the lock opens, it sets off a whole cascade of events. The POAH communicates with the skin (causing sweating), muscles (shivering), blood vessels (opening or closing), respiratory system (panting), and cognition (to find shade or heat). Basically, the whole body and brain get in on the act.

One specific set of events caused by EPs in the POAH is the release of COX enzymes. COX is short for cyclooxygenase. COX enzymes are largely what cause the inflammation part of the immune response. Yes, as we all know, inflammation and pain are critical parts of the immune response. We know the most about two COX enzymes which (surprise, surprise) are called COX-1 and COX-2. Without getting into too much detail about what COX-1 and COX-2 do, let's focus on the fact that they make the fatty acid prostaglandin E2 (PGE2). PGE2 does many things, but we'll focus on how it helps increase and decrease inflammation.

Feeling the Fever

We briefly mentioned this part of the fever mechanism in chapter four when we talked about how PGE2 is given the most credit for increasing the body's thermal set point during a fever. This is where the action happens! In humans, it takes about two hours for all the chemicals to buzz about doing their thing and for us to get to this point.

There's a different time frame for each animal that has been tested. Pigeons have a very delayed fever response. They also have a high normal body temperature—about

43 degrees Celsius.[56] That's interesting because they eat a lot of crap, right? They go for discarded, moldy food scraps and bits of garbage, and who knows what else. If their normal body temperature wasn't so high, they'd likely be sick all the time. Pigeons are so hot, though, that many bacteria just can't live in them.

But back to humans. Back to you. It's been two hours since your dramatic surfing accident, and it's now that PGE2 hits that teeny, tiny part of the brain, *shifts the thermal set point up*, and you start to actually feel a fever coming on. You start getting hot—pigeon hot. You find a bed, turn off the lights, get under the covers, and fever.

Things get interesting here. The fever temperature range is so important because it's where many bacteria and other invaders just can't survive. But it's also where this biochemical orchestra really gets grooving. It's pretty cool to see this in a Petri dish. The higher temperature makes your body produce a crazy amount of white blood cells, which help fight the bad guy invaders. When you look at these white blood cells and their cytokine messengers under a microscope sitting at 36 to 37 degrees, they're like slugs. They're barely moving. They're dead-ish. Okay, that's not a very scientific description, but imagine that's how it looks. Then, you crank the heat to 39.5 degrees, and these things start zipping around, all happy, flexing their muscles and stuff. They're hungry. They're moving and singing. They're *active*. That's why the body is so desperate to get your temperature up there, and it goes into overdrive to make it happen.

IL-1 makes you feel achy, suppresses your appetite, and promotes sleep. IL-1 is a big part of the reason that you just want to lie around sleeping and binge-watching Netflix. The body does this on purpose because it doesn't want you running around, going to work, and playing tennis during a fever. It can't afford the calories for that! I know I've said it before, but the numbers just amaze me: For every degree your temperature increases, your basal metabolic rate increases by 10 to 12.5 percent. So, when you have a four-degree Celsius rise, which can happen in fever, you're burning 40 to 50 percent more energy than usual. So, the body says, "Hey, you gotta lie down because I'm about to use twice as many calories as usual. So, I'm going to make you feel real lousy, to make sure you'll lie down. Okay?"

You get pale and clammy, too, even though you feel like you're burning up inside. This happens because the hypothalamus releases the neurotransmitter *norepinephrine*, which causes vasoconstriction of the blood vessels at the surface. You might remember that's where your blood vessels narrow to force blood to the body's core and decrease heat loss. Of course, later in the fever response, when the set-point and temperature have been adequately raised, the opposite will happen. The blood vessels will open, and you'll sweat to help lower the temperature back to normal.

Just as PGE2 triggered the hypothalamus to release norepinephrine, in turn, norepinephrine triggers the release of another chemical, *acetylcholine*. This has a bunch of responsibilities, including telling the muscles to start shivering. The muscles start contracting and releasing super-fast, which generates heat, helping the body reach the new set point. Acetylcholine activates the burning of *brown fat* to bankroll its energy-expensive goal of shivering. Brown fat is where the body stores extra "insulation." It's the energy you carry around in case of a rainy day. Like now. As well as making you rest, your body taps into the stored energy in brown fat to keep up with the increased caloric demand during fever.

When the body gets into the new set-point temperature of 38.5 to 40.5 degrees Celsius, the baddie bacteria can't survive. As *Pathogenesis of Fever* says, "The induction of fever results in inhibition of bacterial growth, increased bactericidal of neutrophils, production of acute-phase protein synthesis and other physiological changes such as anorexia and somnolence. These changes suggest that fever has an adaptive role in the host's survival during infection."[57] At the fever temperature, bacteria slow down, then die. No more infection. The battle is won! This whole fever mechanism subsides as the body down-regulates EPs and up-regulates endogenous cryogens (ECs)—which do the opposite to their pyrogen buddies and make you cooler. Your temperature drops. You stop shivering. You start feeling normal. The cut on your foot starts to heal, and you get to go surfing again!

Now, as you might have noticed, this whole process is friggin' complicated, and there are other things going on simultaneously—some that we understand well and others we don't fully grasp yet. As the scientist Matthew J. Kluger said, "The stimuli that cause release of cytokines trigger a cascade of responses that have many positive and negative feedback loops, thus making it extremely difficult to determine the precise role of any specific cytokine in fever."[58]

There are other chemicals like RANK and RANKL, which are also released by the key-and-lock mechanism in the POAH, but which we don't absolutely understand right now. EP3 is another chemical triggered by PGE2, which has a receptor in the hypothalamus. We know something is going on there, but we're not 100 percent sure what yet. Yes, there remains much to be learned.

When NSAIDs Interfere

When we interrupt the fever process by taking an NSAID, we interfere with the COX and PGE2 mechanism. Remember how COX enzymes create PGE2, which gets the most credit for raising the thermal set point? *This* is the main target for NSAIDs. Although the various NSAIDs act in nuanced ways, they all inhibit COX enzymes. When you take an NSAID, when EPs float up to the POAH and put their keys in the locks, the COX enzymes just don't get released. The NSAID prevents it. So, you can't make that all-important PGE2, and the thermal set point doesn't get raised. It stays at normal. Then, the mechanism we've spent this chapter discussing doesn't go down.

When you remove one instrument from the orchestra, the whole show gets messed up. Nothing sounds right. It doesn't work anymore. Yes, you feel better. But, you are preventing your immune system from doing its job. How can we expect our immune system to function well, and to help prevent the invaders from gaining entry or being taken care of efficiently if they do enter?

When people feel lousy, achy, tired, hot, inflamed, and miserable, the idea of taking an NSAID and interfering with this process is pretty compelling. They simply want to get rid of the nasty, noxious feeling that comes with fever. On top of that, most people still worry about letting the body do this perfectly orchestrated, incredibly effective, gorgeous fever response. There are also a lot of myths going around that make people nervous or downright fearful. Some of these myths are rooted in truth but have been disproven or distorted over time. Others just aren't true and never have been. In the next chapter, we will look at the most prevalent myths that make people scared of fevers. And I think you're going to be amazed once we break them down.

Chapter Seven: Fever Myths

> *... practitioners often seem to possess an ingrained philosophic opposition towards fever, prompting a knee-jerk response to treat that is not supported by high-level evidence in the ICU population.*
>
> **Dr. Juliet J. Ray and Dr. Carl I. Schulman,**
> **Fever: Suppress It or Let It Ride, 2015**

Blood. Phlegm. Yellow bile. Black bile. That is what the ancient Greeks believed made up the human body. They weren't *entirely* wrong—we each have about 5 litres of blood in us, and for some of us, almost as much phlegm during cold and flu season. But they had no idea about gram-negative bacteria, LPS, cytokines, pyrogens, or cryogens. The Greeks called their four bodily components *humors*, which corresponded to the elements of air, water, fire, and earth. Similar ideas were also developed and documented in civilizations even prior to them, from modern-day India and China, but it was the ancient Greeks, including Hippocrates, who became known in the West for applying the "science" of humors to medicine sometime around 400 BC.[59]

Hippocrates and his followers believed humors flowed through us at all times, keeping the body working well. But if any humor became out of balance, with too much or too little flowing through the body, a fever or other malady would develop. More interesting and relevant than that, they recognized that fever was something *good*. Fevers were the body's way of rejigging these four essential elements. They were a chance to get back in balance. Those ancient Greeks were pretty impressive. Yeah, they had some weird ideas (bloodletting with leeches and purging through vomiting and diarrhea come to mind), but without any of the advantages of modern science, they identified illness, recorded its symptoms, and determined fever was vital to restoring health.

Other ancient peoples had similar insights. There's ample evidence dating back over four thousand years of the same corresponding ideas in India's Ayurveda and Traditional Chinese Medicine (TCM). In fact, these two medical systems continue to teach and treat the elements of fire, earth, metal, water, and wood. The elements must stay in balance amongst the various forces in our bodies, and if they are not, this causes dis-ease. In Ayurveda, using certain dietary, herbal, exercise, physical, and medicinal interventions, the practitioner tries to bring the person back into alignment. In TCM, the doctor may add acupuncture or acupressure to an otherwise similar approach including various lifestyle and medical interventions. Undoubtedly, around the ancient world, doctors were documenting how to manage health conditions given their limited knowledge of the microscopic universe within our bodies.

Today, of course, science has developed far from the understanding of these ancient cultures. We know so much more, and yet misconceptions regarding health and disease are still rampant and commonplace. As far as I know, no one today truly believes the human body only consists of four elements—we get that it's a little more complex—but people do believe completely unproven *and disproven* ideas about many aspects of health and disease, including fever. So, let's look at what these ideas are and why it's been so hard to know the truth from the myths.

Myth: Fever is Bad

The most common misunderstanding here is that fever is bad and must be suppressed. You know my take on this by now, and we've seen the animal and human evidence involved, but I'm going to state it loud and clear: fever is not bad. Fever is good. Yay for fever. However, there's no denying that fever *feels* bad. When someone gets sick, they get aches, chills, sweats, exhaustion, and they think, *Hey, I'm sick. This sucks. I feel lousy.* Then, they mistakenly equate the feeling with the source. The thought goes that fever is making them feel bad, so fever is bad. I understand the connection, and its simplicity is kind of attractive. It's no surprise this has become a widespread belief.

But we've seen that the body is not a simple machine. It's home to an infinite amount of beautiful and complex orchestral processes. Fever feels bad because it is a battle against baddies. Invaders have breached the first few lines of defense, have gained entry, and now our internal army must go through some critical steps and tough times to fight them off. But that doesn't mean we stop fighting. We must persevere and win the battle.

In chapter five I shared a sampling of the clinical data supporting the fact that fever is good. First, R. E. Bryant and his group did a retrospective study on 218 patients with gram-negative bacteremia (which is a type of bacteria in the bloodstream) and found there was a positive correlation between the maximum temperature of the patient on the day of diagnosis and survival.[60] The higher the temperature, the more likely the patient was to survive, and vice versa. Next, that guy Mackowiak published a paper in 1980 where he found a similar relationship between the ability to achieve fever temperatures and the survival from bacterial sepsis in 184 patients.[61] And the last example, M. R. Weinstein's group found that achieving a body temperature of greater than 38 degrees Celsius created a statistically significant higher likelihood of survival in patients with a severe infection called *bacterial peritonitis*.[62]

Myth: Everyone Should Suppress Fevers

That first myth leads to this next one. *If fever is bad, we should stop it, right? Everyone should suppress their fevers.* This idea has been partly fueled by research that shows fever genuinely isn't good for *some* people. There are a handful of cohorts or groups of people whose situations are perhaps worthy of some additional caution when dealing with fever, and there is one—just one—cohort of people whose normal fever process doesn't function properly. A humor has been thrown out of balance, as the ancient Greeks would say. Let's start with the one clear group of concern.

These are people with traumatic brain injuries (TBIs). Tucked behind the forebrain, right next to the visual cortex, is that pea-sized part of the brain called the hypothalamus. If you recall, it is generally regarded the body's primary temperature control centre. And let me tell you: this little nugget of brain matter is incredible. When we get signals from other parts of the body, like the feeling of cold wind on our arms, for example, those signals shoot up to the anterior part of the hypothalamus, which processes the information and sends other signals to the rest of the body to regulate its temperature, in this example by triggering the shivering mechanism. Among many other things, temperature and fever are regulated by this small but mighty part of the brain. It's kind of a big deal.

So, what happens when the hypothalamus gets damaged in a TBI? I'm not talking about when you accidentally open the kitchen cupboard into your head because you weren't paying attention. We're talking about serious brain injuries here, and they can interfere with the hypothalamus's ability to regulate temperature. In this state, it can't tell the fevering body, "Whoa, wait! We've reached the new set point. Time to shut off the pyrogens and crank the cryogens, so things don't get hotter." That doesn't necessarily happen when the hypothalamus is injured, so we can see extreme fevers, even seizures, and other nasty stuff happening. So, if we don't actively suppress fevers in patients with TBIs, they are statistically more likely to have negative outcomes. And we don't want that.

But the key point is that people with TBIs are the *only* population in which there is published clinical evidence of a statistical benefit to interfering with the fever process. These patients should actively suppress their fevers, but that doesn't mean everyone must. And that leads us nicely to our next myth.

Myth: The Same Guidelines Apply to All

Remember the Hippocratic Oath? It inspired the most important guideline for doctors: First, do no harm. That *does* apply to all. Everyone is worthy of the same care and caution in treatments. But the way in which we do no harm and the best methods to help vary based on the individual we are treating, in their particular life stage, with all their history, nuances, preferences, fears, and strengths.

As we think about fever management, it's sensible to apply extra caution to some vulnerable groups. These include very weak and frail patients with an already low body habitus (physique); those with cachexia, which is a metabolic condition in severe and advanced chronic illness; those with pre-existing severe cardiovascular disease; pregnant women; and infants. As we've discussed, fever does increase the body's already significant energy requirements for maintaining temperature. It's calorically incredibly expensive, with a 20 to 50 percent increase in caloric demand. While we know there's no benefit to preventing fever in most, we want to take extra care with those most vulnerable people.

Imagine an elderly patient in hospice care whose body is already not doing well, mostly skin and bone, having not eaten well in weeks or even months, surviving mostly off nutrients delivered through an intravenous drip. They literally cannot afford the calories required to fever. Also, the fever would make them feel awful, when they are already feeling pretty miserable. In cases like this, it probably makes sense for their doctor to suppress their fever by giving them some ASA or ibuprofen. It still might not be medically necessary, and it really is a judgment call for the patient and doctor to make together, but fever suppression probably makes good sense in this situation.

Another vulnerable group are those patients in intensive care units (ICUs). These folks are sick. It used to be that ICU patients were constantly given NSAIDs to prevent fevers from developing. The idea was that they were so weak they couldn't risk getting a fever, as their bodies wouldn't handle it. We now know that's not true.

Paul Young is a fever researcher whose work I'm following with most interest these days. He's an ICU specialist and co-clinical lead at the Wellington Regional Hospital ICU, in New Zealand. In 2015 he conducted The HEAT Trial[63] in which his team gave seven hundred ICU patients with fever either intravenous acetaminophen or an intravenous placebo every six hours until they got better, were discharged, or died. They measured the number of ICU-free days each person had—that is, days they were alive and didn't need to be in the ICU anymore—within a 28-day period. What happened? The group who got the acetaminophen did *not* have improved outcomes over the placebo group. The drug didn't help them get out of ICU faster. In fact, patients in the placebo group were released from ICU, on average, one day earlier than the acetaminophen group. That detail is not statistically significant enough to imply that the acetaminophen made things worse, but the results do confirm that *it doesn't improve outcomes* for ICU patients. It simply doesn't help them get home sooner.

In 2019, Paul Young then published The REACTOR Trial,[64] a randomized controlled trial on 184 adults who were in the ICU, deeply sedated with no response to voice, had a fever, and were mechanically ventilated—as in, a machine was helping them breathe. I think it's fair to call this a vulnerable group. Young's team split the participants into a *fever treatment* group and an *ignore the fever* group. Of the 89 patients in the *fever treatment* group, 23 died in the ICU. In the *ignore the fever* group, 23 of the 89 patients also died in the ICU. The same. Again, there were no statistically significant differences between these two groups in ICU-free days or in their ninety-day survival rates. Nothing. Bubkas.

As we can see, it's not so cut-and-dry that we can apply one guideline to all people or even all people in the most vulnerable groups. Paul Young's studies were on a population in whom managing fever has always *just been done*. It has been accepted practice. It is where fever management should matter the most and make the biggest difference. Yet research proves it doesn't.

Myth: Fever Causes Seizures

You might have heard the myth that fevers can induce seizures in babies and that proves fever is bad. Seizures *have* been reported in infants with fevers, so naturally, we want to explore any connection.

Here's the deal with infants: they have immature thermo-regulatory systems. Their ability to control their temperature isn't fully developed, and it makes sense. They were hanging out in a beautiful, constantly warmed womb for nine months, then they enter the world and suddenly have to deal with all these new environmental changes. For the first time in their development, they have to regulate their temperature. It takes some time to get the hang of it.

In N. Paul Rosman's paper assessing febrile seizures (which is just a medical term for *fever with seizures*), he points out that, "In the child who convulses with fever, it is always important to consider that something in addition to the fever has caused the child to have a seizure." So, the fever itself isn't the cause of the problem—there's something else going on, and it's important to find out what. Possible causes of febrile seizures include meningitis or encephalitis, systemic illness, head trauma, intoxication, electrolyte imbalance, low blood sugar, or a phakomatoses (a type of genetic or acquired disorder). It is *most* important to rule out meningitis or encephalitis as these must be treated… or things can go bad.

You have to treat the underlying problem, not just the fever. In fact, in the infant population, research has proven that giving NSAIDs to manage fevers has no impact on febrile seizure activity.[65] As Mackowiak says, "Unfortunately, antipyretic therapy has not been shown to protect against recurrences of febrile seizure in the few controlled trials that have been conducted to date."[66] If the baby is going to have a seizure, it will happen whether or not you give them NSAIDs. Trying to stop it by only lowering the fever just doesn't work. The key is to find and treat the underlying cause of the fever. So, although it used to be common practice to give febrile infants NSAIDs, that's not necessarily best practice anymore. We still want to protect our babies from seizures and other scary stuff, but we now know NSAIDs are not necessarily the way in which to do it.

Myth: Fever Is the Body Losing Control of Its Temperature

There was once the idea that fever was safe up until 40.5 degrees Celsius, and beyond that, it could cause damage. This led to the fear that if you let a fever ride, it would continue beyond the safe zone, and you'd be in trouble, so it was better to be proactive and bring the fever down immediately.

Fever does not typically go higher than 40.5 degrees.[67,68,69] If someone has a temperature beyond that, they likely have hyperthermia, which is an entirely different issue. That's uncontrolled heating of the body. Fever is well-controlled, and we don't need to fear it escalating further. It just won't happen.

Myth: Fever Prevents Healing

Here's how this one goes: Fever puts stress on the body, and that stress prevents or delays healing. Sounds logical, right? But yet again, there is little to no evidence to support this theory. And I mean as far as I have been able to discern, like no evidence in the history of peer-reviewed medical research. (The only exception, as we've discussed, is with TBI patients.)

Instead, as we've seen, fever is an essential part of the healing process. It's integral to the immune response. Incredibly, the human body can often heal without being allowed to fever, but it's like forcing Novak Djokovic to play tennis with his left hand. He'll still hit the ball, but it won't be the world's best game. Remember the studies we discussed in chapter five on rhinovirus, chickenpox, measles, and septicemia? They showed that suppressing fevers means staying sick for longer. It forces your body to fight these infections with a handicapped immune system.

Myth: Animal Studies Don't Tell Us about Fever in Humans

Remember all that stuff I told you back in chapter three about fever throughout the animal kingdom? In addition to all the human studies we've looked at since, we saw that when animals are not allowed to let their fevers ride, they die. Yet, humans do not die when we suppress our fevers. So, the misbelief says: We can't draw helpful knowledge from animal studies as they are too different from humans. The results of suppressing fevers aren't the same.

It's smart to ask questions about how animal research should impact our understanding of human experiences. Let's break it down. Why do we even test on animals? Well, for starters the types of studies that are run on animals would not pass ethical standards for human research. You just can't do the things they can to animals, to people. Animal models allow for extreme conditions to be tested. Animal models are able to be given equivalently more NSAIDS under well-controlled test conditions. They're exposed to prolonged extreme temperatures. They're subjected to all sorts of stressors that human testing cannot and should not do. This has been done so we can understand what happens under extreme circumstances. In turn, this lets us unravel the many complicated processes involved.

Animals die when they can't fever because their temperature is suppressed *far more aggressively* than for a human who pops a couple of pills. But the processes are largely the same. Animal studies provide us with the gift of insights we just can't determine in more regulated human experiences.

And don't forget... we're not just relying on animal studies to inform our understanding of fever. There is a solid base of human clinical data, and we've already talked about some of them. Again, go back to chapter five if you want to re-examine some of the compelling studies. Use the citations listed at the end of this book to find the relevant references.

What Next?

We've come a long way in our journey of understanding fever. We've established what happens during a fever and that it truly feels crappy. We know fever occurs throughout the animal kingdom, and it's a survival mechanism that continues to thrive through life on earth. We know what happens when we interrupt fever by taking NSAIDs and why it's so tempting, even though there's no evidence to support it. We've seen that suppressing fever means staying sick for longer, and we've discussed the most common myths and misconceptions about fever.

Now we understand what we're working with, how can we actually work *with* fever? When we're confident we don't need to suppress it, we can explore how to benefit from fever. We don't just need to put up with fever; we can actually harness it for good. And this isn't a new idea. Fever as a therapy has been used for a long time with sometimes incredible results. In the next chapter, we'll look at some of these examples and explore how we can benefit from the body's natural systems.

Chapter Eight: Benefitting from the Body's Natural Systems

Now, as each of the parts of the body, like every other instrument, is for the sake of some purpose, viz. some action, it is evident that the body as a whole must exist for the sake of some complex action.

Aristotle, philosopher, circa 1550

In 1891, a sick and terminally ill Italian immigrant named Monsignore Zola stumbled into the New York Hospital with a large, cancerous tumour.[70] This thing was impossible to miss. It was sticking out the side of his neck, still under the skin, and the size of egg. An egg. You'll want to see this thing.[71] I imagine Mr. Zola must've been freaking out.

At the time, radiotherapy and chemotherapy hadn't been developed, let alone immunotherapy. Surgery was the treatment of the day. Zola had already had two operations at other hospitals which were clearly *not* successful in controlling the cancer, now in his right tonsil. At this point, his expected survival was likely weeks or perhaps months. Things must have seemed hopeless. But, enter Dr. William Bradley Coley, a Harvard class of 1888 graduate working as a surgeon at New York Hospital (now Memorial Sloan Kettering Hospital).

Just the previous year, in the fall of 1890, Coley had treated seventeen-year-old Elisabeth Dashiell, the "adopted sister" of John D. Rockefeller Junior. Dashiell had a very painful, swollen right hand due to a sarcoma (cancer of soft tissues and bone), ultimately requiring amputation below her elbow. Sadly, the surgery was too late. The tumours had already grown into her breasts, lymph nodes, and liver. Dashiell suffered severe pain requiring escalating doses of morphine until she sadly died of liver failure from advanced disease on January 23, 1891.[72]

Coley was, as the story goes, profoundly impacted by Dashiell's death. By day, he continued performing surgeries; by night, he poured through his hospital's sarcoma case files, hunting for a cure for the cancer that killed her. He found about ninety case reports of other patients with sarcomas, forty-seven of which were well-documented with long-term follow up.[73] While trawling through these cases, one particular report on a German immigrant, Fred Stein, caught his eye.

In 1884, Stein was diagnosed with a sarcoma of his cheek. The guy went through four surgeries to treat it, and they were all unsuccessful. Just to kick him while he was down, late that year he also developed a severe post-operative *erysipelas* infection from the fever-causing bacteria *Streptococcus pyogenes*. There were no antibiotics at that time, and erysipelas was a serious skin infection that often caused death. However, in Stein's case, when the fever broke and left, so too did his tumours and enlarged lymph nodes. Dr. Bull, his attending physician, witnessed all visible signs of the tumours disappear along with the skin infection. Stein was discharged from hospital cancer-free in 1885.

Five months after Dashiell's death, Coley (after nothing short of an extraordinary effort) tracked Stein down in New York's Lower East Side. Stein agreed to let Coley and Bull examine and photograph him back in hospital, and the doctors found no residual cancer.[74] None.

The Soiled Bandage Experiment

At some point in Coley's hunt for a cure for sarcoma, he came across work done twenty years earlier by the German professor Dr. Wilhelm Busch, who published a case report in the March. 23, 1868 edition of the medical journal *Berliner Klinische Wochenschrift*.[75] Busch reported observing a head and neck cancer "resorb" after an erysipelas infection in one of his patients. He suspected the erysipelas and its resulting fever caused the cancer's resorption.

Busch put this observation to the test when a nineteen-year-old girl with a large sarcoma on her face entered his clinic on the same day a man with a severe case of erysipelas (a skin infection) walked through his doors. Ah-ah! So, this girl presents with a giant tumour on her head and neck region. It's bad. She can't breathe properly, and her eye won't close right. Meanwhile, her bedmate is covered in bandages trying to patch up his leaking erysipelas lesions, and Busch seizes the opportunity. Could he actually artificially create a "spontaneous remission" like he previously saw? What if he took the disgusting dressings covered in puss and blood and a buttload of *S. pyogenes*, and smeared them all over the young girl's tumour? And you know where this is going... he actually did it. Mind-blowing. Imagine a doctor trying that now. At the very least, their license to practice would be bye bye, for life.

Busch burned a small area of skin over the girl's tumour and placed a soiled, puss-filled bandage taken directly from the man's festering erysipelas lesion. As expected, she got really, really sick, just like her bedmate. She developed a rash and she fevered. Busch monitored her, kept her comfortable, and I'm sure prayed to dear god that his idea wouldn't hurt her. *But it started to work*. Sure as shootin', as she developed high fevers of 40 degrees Celsius and some classic erysipelas, her large tumour shrank and softened with impressive speed, allowing her to breathe and close her eye again. Here's the kicker, though: When the erysipelas resolved, the tumour slowly started to grow back, growing to its original size within a month. Busch was watching a true-life example of the power of fever therapy.

Forty-Seven Spontaneous Surprises

Coley learned to read and write German during his university studies, allowing him to read the reports of Busch and another German scientist, Friedrich Fehleisen, who published reports in 1882 detailing the added sophistication of actually culturing the bacteria and injecting it into patients. Yes, you read that right. He collected and then successfully grew *S. pyogenes*, then injected it into patients with cancer. Fehleisen published the outcomes of his initial study injecting live cultured *S. Pyogenes* into seven advanced cancer patients, impressively achieving remissions in three of them.[76]

In total, Coley found forty-seven cases of "disappearance of malignancies during an erysipelas attack" in the hospital records—cases where cancer patients got a fever, then the cancer disappeared.[77] Sounds crazy, right? These were referred to as "spontaneous" remissions, which to him seemed a little unfair, or at least not very insightful. It suggested these cancers vanished all of a sudden, with no explanation. Poof. But in fact, Coley thought he knew a bit more about what went down in those instances. And thanks to his efforts, we now do too.

In each of these cases, the patient had a confirmed cancer diagnosis, their disease was advanced (metastatic), and could not be managed with surgery alone. Every patient happened to get an infection, which caused a fever, and when that fever broke the cancer disappeared, and doctors confirmed a remission. This occurred in every one of these forty-seven cases that Coley uncovered in just two years of research. And remember, this was the 1800s, and Coley was searching in person through physical records in his spare time. Imagine what he might've found with more time, electronic access to vast databases, and the all-knowing PubMed.

Coley in Action

Now, remember that poor guy, Monsignore Zola, with the egg-sized tumour and two failed surgeries? He entered New York Hospital right as Coley was fresh-off chasing down Fred Stein, and reading the reports of Busch, Fehleisen, and others showing cancer remissions after fevers caused by *S. pyogenes*. Here was Coley's chance. Coley and his colleagues prepared bacterial cultures, applied them to Zola's open wounds, and injected them into the tumour. But they couldn't create an infection strong enough to enduce a fever. Coley tried a fresh specimen in a larger dose, and within two hours Zola got chills, a headache, and vomiting, but his temperature only hit a maximum of 39 degrees Celsius. Still, the tumour shrank for a month, but then started to worsen again.

By this time, Coley was able to procure a fresh *S. pyogenes* culture from one of the world's top bacteriologists of the day, Robert Koch in Berlin. Within one hour of injection of this fresh *S. pyogenes*, Zola's temperature rose above 40 Celsius and he was very sick with pain and vomiting. The nightmare-ish infection lasted two weeks, and by the end, the neck tumour was gone. Zola survived the cancer *and* the nasty skin infection. Coley probably breathed a sigh of relief, cracked a beer to celebrate, and went on to treat nine more patients, the results of which he published in *The American Journal of the Medical Sciences*.[78] Unfortunately, he was only able to mount a fever in two of those cases, presumably because the cultures he used were not potent enough. Interestingly though, in those two patients who mounted a fever, the cancer resolved in one, and there was a partial response in the other. Zola remained in good health when Coley saw him four years later. Reportedly, he died eight years after his fever treatment in Italy of unknown causes.

Fever Therapy Evolution

Coley's work was an early type of fever therapy. The phrase *fever therapy* means deliberately using fever as a treatment, and that's exactly what Coley did. As Matthew Kluger explained decades later, "[N]umerous studies have demonstrated that small elevations in body temperature, similar to those observed during fever, enhance the immune response."[79] Coley wasn't the first doctor to have this idea, but you'll soon see why he's the most famous for it.

Before we get to that, though, I know what you're thinking: We don't use fever therapies in this way today, so what gives? Cancer patients aren't lining up to get slathered with other people's dirty bandages. If Coley's research was so compelling and his treatment so successful, what happened, and why aren't we using fever therapies now? Come follow the trail of fever therapies with me, and I'll explain all.

We have a good understanding of Coley's studies thanks, largely, to his daughter, Helen Coley Nauts. After his death, she started the nonprofit Cancer Research Institute and properly documented her father's work. It needed her help because organization was not Coley's forté, and his own records were a little hard to follow. In fact, he really didn't do the best job with his studies. I mean, the guy so was insightful, and learning about his work is like watching art in action. But like art, it was a bit messy.

From Helen's incredible work, though, we get a great picture of what happened. After Zola, Coley treated those nine patients but struggled to get them all to mount fevers. He then tried to make the bacterial cultures stronger and in higher doses, and tragically, two patients died consecutively. Then, Coley switched up the method, using dead bacteria instead of live versions in order to avoid fatalities ever again. This made the process safer, but the fevers weren't quite as strong, which meant remissions weren't as drastic. But, you know, at least more patients didn't die as a result of the treatment itself. Which is kind of most important.

Then, Coley started using other bugs in addition to *S. pyogenes* and created cocktails of three or four different bacteria. This is where his documentation got even more squiffy, and we really owe Helen some more thanks. Coley was creating bacterial concoctions of all kinds of formulas and strengths. Sometimes they caused fevers, sometimes they didn't, and it wasn't always clear why because the experimentation was kind of haphazard. They certainly didn't follow current standard research practices. However, he narrowed down a selection of bacterial cocktails that included extracts of *S. pyogenes* and *Serratia marcescens (Bacillus prodigiosus)* and named them Coley's Toxins. That name is now famous—though admittedly, only in the world of fever therapies.

Between 1891 and 1896, Coley published sixteen papers on his treatment method, and at least forty-two other physicians published reports on positive outcomes in their own patients treated with Coley's Toxins. Over the course of his career, Coley treated about one thousand patients with inoperable and advanced cancers, with many achieving complete or partial remissions. He noted the patients who had the best fevers got the best results. Those that did not develop a fever from the bacterial injections did not have responses in their cancers. In most of his cancer patients, Coley used a combination of surgery, his toxins, and, when it came around in the early 1900s, radiotherapy.

In 1992, Charlie O. Starnes published *Coley's Toxins in Perspective* in the journal *Nature*, where he identified 170 of those patients whose cancer was inoperable and who received *only* Coley's Toxins—no surgery or radiation.[80] He found a remission rate of 64 percent with a five-year survival rate of 44 percent. That's super impressive by any standard in the world of oncology. Then and now. But as you may not have heard of this cancer treatment before, you know this isn't the end of Coley's story. Before we get there, though, let's take a detour to Europe.

More Fever Therapy Discoveries

In Russia between 1946 and 1953, Dr. Nina Klyuyeva did similar work with a tropical parasite called *Trypanosoma cruzi*, which causes Chaga's Disease. For those of us in the northern hemisphere, this parasite is no big deal, but it's endemic in Latin America, infecting about nine million people per year.[81] Like *S. pyogenes*, *T. cruzi* creates a fever response. In one of Klyuyeva's books, she describes thirty-two cases of patients with cancer treated with fever therapy.[82] It's a detailed account including images of tumours, laboratory data, and detailed descriptions. Of those thirty-two patients, twenty-one were reportedly cured by this treatment.

Again, a correlation was found between those who developed a fever from the parasite and those who experienced remission. The better the fever, the better the result. It was a small study, but that too is a compelling result that requires further discussion and enquiry. If these sorts of findings are found to be reproducible, we need to explore how and why, now.

I also have to mention the work of Julius Wagner-Jauregg, an Austrian psychiatrist who won the Nobel Prize in Medicine in 1927. A big part of me doesn't want to mention him (you'll soon understand why), but his work and notoriety warrant inclusion in a thorough discussion of the power of fever. Juaregg came from Austro-Hungarian nobility, sporting the most pompous mustache, like Agatha Christie's Detective Poirot. As I've eluded to, he was a bit of an ass, to put it mildly. He applied to join the Nazi party but was rejected, despite the fact, and because his first wife was Jewish. He went on to support eugenics and forcibly sterilizing those with mental illness. Not a good guy.

But apparently, he was clever or well-funded enough to act on others' good ideas. He became famous for promoting a unique and immunologic approach to treating mental illnesses. What did this guy do to be honoured with such a grand award as the Nobel Prize? He purposely infected folks with malaria. Not in a crazy bad guy way, but in a Coley way.[83]

In his clinic in Vienna, he worked with many patients with syphilis. Back then, there weren't any antibiotics effective against syphilis, and if left untreated and allowed to go into its third and final stage, syphilis would get into the central nervous system, causing neurosyphilis. Symptoms of neurosyphilis include meningitis, stroke, paralysis, dementia, and psychosis. In Wagner-Jauregg's time, neurosyphilis was rapidly rising in incidence, leading to tons of hospitalizations for psychosis and paralysis. In fact, about 10 percent of all psychiatric admissions at the time were because of neurosyphilis.

This is where Wagner-Jauregg's idea came in. Okay, fine, it wasn't actually *his* idea. (As though I'm not thrilled to pop his unwarranted prize glory.) The psychiatrist Alexander Rosenblum from Ukraine had already reported treating thirty-two patients with psychosis using malaria, typhoid, and relapsing fever, curing sixteen of them. *When?* you ask. In 1876. Half a century before Wagner-Jauregg received his Nobel Prize. But Rosenblum's findings were published in an obscure journal, and never gained widespread notoriety.

Wagner-Jauregg had been researching fever therapies like Coley's Toxins, and in 1917, he started experimenting with his own version of *S. pyogenes* for psychosis. He also tried tuberculin injections mixed with iodine-mercury. After thirty years of experimentation, he finally tried injecting the malaria parasite *Plasmodium vivax* into syphilis patients. He chose that particular bug because it was the least aggressive option that also produced prolonged, high, and recurring fevers. It also gave him the option to follow the malarial treatment with quinine if he needed to treat and stop the malaria.

The process was certainly risky with as many as 15 percent of patients dying. Remember, quinine was the only treatment back then, today this would be different. But an impressive 30 percent of the patients had their otherwise untreatable neurosyphilis (and malaria) cured. Obviously, we don't want patients dying from their treatments, and there are reasons this process isn't used anymore. Wagner-Jauregg continued his malaria treatment until 1940, but as far as I know, it hasn't been done since. His risky technique wasn't the ideal cure for syphilis, as in the end antibiotics came to the rescue. But it did once again tell us something essential. By using a fever-inducing infection, you can often overcome chronic infections, advanced cases of neurological diseases, and even advanced cancers.

What About the 21st Century?

There have been many more reported cases with similar findings published over past decades, but I want to share one of the most recent and relevant cases from 2020. It involved a man with widespread, very advanced Hodgkin lymphoma (cancer of the lymph nodes).[84] He'd lost a lot of weight, had end-stage renal failure, and was now on dialysis. PET scans showed numerous large tumours and lymph nodes from his neck, throughout his chest and abdomen, and into his pelvis and groin. Not long after being diagnosed with Stage 3B disease, this man started getting breathless and wheezy. He'd developed a severe case of COVID-19. He was in the hospital for eleven days receiving life-saving treatment before being sent home. While in hospital, he was sick with a high fever that lasted for days. Four months later, when he had his next PET scan, the lymphoma had disappeared. It was just gone.

This guy hadn't had any steroids or chemotherapy. He got an infection, had a fever, and his tumours disappeared. His medical team published the details in the *British Journal of Haematology*, saying, "We hypothesise that the SARS-CoV-2 [COVID-19] infection triggered an anti-tumour immune response, as has been described with other infections ...." Fascinating, right?

The War on Cancer

But let's get back to our story. In the late 1800s, Coley had success using fevers to dissolve cancerous tumours. In the 1920s, Wagner-Jauregg got a Nobel Prize for inducing malaria fevers to treat chronic disease. Then what? The next major milestone came in 1971, when President Nixon stood in front of the American flag and all his people and declared war on cancer.

Cancer was the United States' second leading cause of death, and in signing the new National Cancer Act into law, Nixon propelled a huge amount of money and interest into finding "a cure for cancer." The impact stretched beyond America as industry and clinical communities worldwide collaborated and built on each other's work.

However, Coley's Toxins didn't get any of this gorgeous new research money because just a few years earlier, in 1965, it was *discredited* by the United States Food and Drug Administration (FDA). Yeah. And it was added to the Unproven Methods of Cancer Management list by the American Cancer Society. They didn't like Coley's haphazard research methods, and that's fair. Science must be conducted in a more controlled manner to be considered reliable.

Coley's Toxins were far from a perfect treatment but talk about throwing the baby out with the bath water. When the FDA discredited Coley's Toxins, it had the unfortunate effect of making people believe the treatment had *nothing* of value. Instead of going back to the drawing board and trying to improve on Coley's exciting discoveries, the pharmaceutical and oncology communities dropped Coley's Toxins totally, in favour of other, newer treatments like chemotherapy. I understand how and why this happened, but it was a real shame—especially because the FDA removed that classification a decade later. They went back on what they'd said, and they now allow Coley's Toxins to be used as an "investigational new drug." Which basically means it's not approved for general, free-for-all use, but it can be applied for in clinical trials.

With Coley's Toxins out of the picture—at least for the time being—chemotherapy became the research golden child, and it showed excellent results.

See, when an oncologist puts a person onto a cancer treatment program, they'll start with a snapshot of the person's health status. They'll order scans of the relevant areas, take blood tests, and conduct a physical exam to get an overall picture of what's going on. Typically, they will take another clinical snapshot after three or more months of treatment, hoping to see significant improvements in all these parameters. Over time, research clearly showed no other treatment resulted in a faster or bigger improvement in these snapshots than chemotherapy. Like radiotherapy, chemotherapy makes tumours shrink or disappear faster than anything else ever did.

However, chemotherapy and radiotherapy are cytotoxic, which means they poison living cells—healthy and unhealthy ones alike. They don't just kill cancer cells; they also kill the rapidly dividing "self" cells, too. Here's what happens: All cells in the body create copies of themselves all the time. You grow millions of skin cells a day, for example. The lining of your digestive system regenerates so fast that it is basically brand new every few days. Hair follicles readily grow and replace themselves. (Well, for most people)

You've seen pictures of DNA, right, with the two strands entwined around each other like a twisted ladder? Those two strands of DNA are inside every cell. When the cell copies itself, it zips open and unwinds these strands, makes duplicates of each of them, then twists itself back up again. So, each strand is now two strands, making two cells with DNA from the one cell with DNA. I mean, it's a little more technical than that, but that's essentially what happens. When chemotherapy or radiation comes along, while the two strands of DNA are unzipped and actively unwinding or rewinding, they damage the DNA beyond repair. They kill the DNA, killing the cell, so it can't make more and more copies of itself (which is what cancer is).

But since they target all cells undergoing the unzipping, unwinding, rewinding process—healthy cells as well as the nasty, cancerous ones—they cause our good stuff to die too. The most rapidly dividing healthy cells include the bone marrow, hair follicles, skin, nails, and lining of the digestive tract, amongst others. This explains why those undergoing chemotherapy and radiotherapy frequently have low blood counts, hair loss, skin and nail changes, nausea, vomiting, and diarrhea. Their guts can't replenish their cells fast enough. Hair follicles can't rebuild fast enough. The side effects of chemotherapy and radiation can be rough.

People feel bad, but yes, their tumours do get smaller. That's exciting. For many people, that's life saving. Chemotherapy and radiotherapy can be *incredible* in that respect.

It wasn't just these two treatments that gobbled up the research money and attention. I've talked about them because it's such a major factor for many people, but in the years following Nixon's declaration of war, lots of other ideas took the medical research spotlight, including DNA, gene therapy, and the Human Genome Project to name a few. They all brought exciting, wonderful discoveries, but it unfortunately came at the cost of fever therapy.

Searching for A Better Cancer Treatment

Say you were using the ultimate version of Coley's Toxins that meet the requirements to become approved for use today. Going through all the phases of widely accepted robust clinical trials. A formula safe enough that it doesn't kill patients, can be used long enough to get results, yet is strong enough to build a robust fever reaction.

Now, say you took snapshots of your health status before treatment and three months in, which, as mentioned, is fairly standard practice when treating people with cancer. These snapshots are an assessment of how a treatment is going. It measures the result of a treatment from one time to the next. When a person goes from one scan to the next 3 months later and there has been no progression of their disease, this we call *progression-free survival* (PFS). This is not the same as *overall survival* (OS), which measures how long a patient lives from the time of their cancer diagnosis. Most studies on treatments today look at PFS, as it is simply easier to measure (time and money) that OS. It's also, I guess, human nature and a scientific preference to measure success from one point in time to another. So, what would PFS tell us if we were to compare the effects of chemotherapy and fever therapy? You'd likely see better results quicker with chemo than with the fever therapy.

That might surprise you after hearing me bang on about Coley's Toxins all chapter. But here's why it's true *and still interesting*: Coley's original fever therapy work showed some fast and full responses, but he was pumping those patients with two to three weekly or daily injections at times. He was also using doses that were strong enough to cause serious fevers, but it also did end up killing people. That is why the subsequent versions were safer than Coley's original treatments, but at the same time making them way less effective. The late versions didn't destroy tumours in a single fever event like Zola experienced. The results certainly won't be as good as you'd see with the equivalent length of chemo and radiotherapy treatments.

But Coley's Toxins show us there's real promise for a treatment that works by stimulating the immune system to fight the cancer. It would also do so without all of the side effects of chemotherapy and radiation, that can oh so negatively impact people's quality of life. A safe and effective fever therapy would likely require multiple treatments over a longer period of time. With the exception of the periodic fever responses, which would undoubtedly feel lousy and suck, this approach wouldn't be near as toxic as most treatments. I suspect that fever therapy may ultimately yield better results where it really matters, in OS. Maybe the PFS results wouldn't be as good, but the OS might be better.

We'll look more at cancer survival rates in chapter ten, but here's what I want you to take away from this chapter: Fever therapies like *S. pyogenes*, Coley's Toxins, Klyuyeva's *Trypanosoma cruzi*, Wagner-Jauregg's malarial *Plasmodia vivax*, and the work of others I haven't had space to mention here are all *so* promising, but none of them were ready for prime time. Given the scientific and technological advancements of today, we can see these seemingly disparate approaches share the common thread of fever. There is critical and essential knowledge to be gained from studying this defense response that has been perfected over four hundred million years. That is what binds all these approaches together.

Surely, we can develop a treatment to stimulate fever in a safe and effective way. In the last chapter of this book, I'll share my hypothesis around this, which I'm hoping to do research on. But we're not quite there yet. We don't have a standardized fever therapy treatment that's safe, effective, and less destructive than chemotherapy and radiotherapy. It's not likely to come in any way Coley could've imagined, but it is coming because fever therapy is evolving.

I also want to foreshadow our upcoming discussion on how these ideas have morphed into the new and rapidly developing field of *immunotherapy*, which simply means a treatment that uses the immune system. Sounds like fever therapy, right? Since fever is an integral part of the immune response. But this modern imagining of fever therapies is more targeted, more intelligent, and less atomic bomb-like than anything Coley and his contemporaries cooked up. In the next chapter, we'll look at what immunotherapies can do for you, me, and all of us.

Chapter Nine: The Evolution of Fever Therapy into Modern Immunotherapy

If indeed any were so good a physician as to be able to produce fever, it would not be necessary to look for any other remedy in sickness.

Rufus of Ephesus, Greek physician and author, circa 100

By now, it is abundantly clear that fever is an ancient, incredibly intelligent and orchestrated event involving much of the body and innumerable cells. Nature would have us believe that fever is highly effective in helping the immune system win battles, since much of the animal kingdom uses this mechanism for its survival. Nonetheless, as evidenced by stories like that of our dear Dr. William Coley, finding a reasonably well-tolerated treatment that effectively kicks the body into a fever has proven difficult. For one thing, it seems to take quite a load of live bugs to do it. This, of course, makes the patient feel horrible. And there's the potential harm of creating an infectious situation that can get out of hand, even with powerful antibiotics and other treatments available today. But there is hope. Over the past century plus, the knowledge gained from fever therapy has led to incredible advancements in immunotherapy.

In the last chapter, I said that immunotherapy is a type of treatment that uses the immune system, but it's more accurate to say that these treatments target and adjust specific aspects of the immune system, allowing or promoting it to do the work of attacking the invader. As we'll discuss in this chapter, the immunotherapy drugs and treatments that have been developed to date have been targeted to one particular cell, cytokine (chemical messenger), or mechanism (checkpoints) of the immune system.

We've really come a long way in our understanding of the immune system in the last few decades. The timeline for the most significant fever-related immunotherapy discoveries is very interesting. There was relatively little research in this space for most of the 19th and 20th centuries, with sporadic advancements. However, since the turn of the 21st century, the scientific and medical communities have rapidly accelerated research in this field. In 2000 a USA survey showed that of the $104 billion spent on cancer research, vaccines or immunotherapeutic agents featured prominently among the almost 400 anticancer products under development."[85] There's been nothing short of exponential growth since then. In 2020 alone, the FDA approved fifteen new immunotherapy treatments.

But let's take a quick look back to when things started getting exciting. In 1991, Pierre van der Bruggen published a landmark paper that identified a specific protein or antigen (Ag) on melanoma cells that could be recognized by the immune system. Specifically, these could be found by those T-cells, the white blood cells that hunts out foreign invaders. Remember in chapter six we talked about cytotoxic T-lymphocytes (CTLs), the trained cancer killers that remember their targets? If these T-cells could be trained to recognize and attack specific targets, like Bruggen's melanoma Ags, that could change the cancer treatment landscape forever. His paper rekindled a widespread interest into immunotherapy research and development. There are now several other tumour-specific Ags that have been recognized and cloned in labs around the world. This exciting work continues today.

Next, the research community shifted its gaze to optimizing the immune responses with these Ags to leverage them to treat cancer. Another landmark paper published in 2001 in *Nature* by Robert Schreiber and Lloyd Old's group demonstrated that lymphocytes and interferon-gamma (IFNg is one of those cytokines or messengers) have anti-tumour effects, even in mice without functional immune systems.[86] Lymphocytes are those Pac-man cells that are always looking for invaders to gobble up. IFNg is one of the cytokines that Ag-stimulated lymphocytes produce to signal the rest of the immune system on what to do next. This was a particularly important finding as some previous studies had indicated lymphocytes were not effective at cancer immunosurveillance, and interest in this important immune function had waned. Rekindled.

Schrieber and Old (huge fan of their work) also suggested that by the time the immune system finds a cancer, it no longer recognizes the cancer cells as foreign, allowing the cancer cells to escape the immune system. Doh! So then, research had to dig into how to assist the immune system's recognition and response against these cell-specific Ags, and into preventing the cancer cells from disguising themselves. Not a small task.

Over the past couple of decades, the research into all this stuff has exploded. Another topic of interest in this world has more to do with how tumours try to outsmart these immune defenses. In this particular case, how it tricks the immune system. A fabulous paper by Corthay[87] helps further develop our understanding of how tumours send signals out into the body to subvert and hide from the immune system's defense response.[88]

We have also learned a great deal more about the various cytokines involved in the immune response against bugs and cancer. Each of these topics and more importantly, how they work together in an immune response, has led to the discovery of today's major immunotherapy approaches. The immunotherapy repertoire now includes four major classes of treatments: *checkpoint inhibitors, adoptive cell therapies, therapeutic vaccines, and non-specific immune-modulating agents.* Together, these approaches are spearheading the future of cancer care. Yes, I know, most of the examples in this chapter are about cancer, simply because that's the world I work in. It also happens to be the space in which much of the research has been done, despite the fact that immunotherapy is also used to treat many other diseases. So, what exactly are these four types of immunotherapy approaches? I'm so glad you asked.

Checkpoint Inhibitors

Checkpoints put the brakes on the immune system, particularly those cancer killing T-cells. You don't want your immune system going hog-wild every hour of the day without any checks and balances. Once the immune system is turned on to do good work, it must then be turned off before it starts doing some bad work, as happens to people with autoimmune diseases. Their immune system gets way over-zealous, starting and not stopping, attacking everything—including parts of its own healthy body.

To try and prevent that kind of mayhem, the body has checkpoints to control the immune response. T-cells have receptors on them that act as breaks, and when our healthy cells want to turn those T-cells off, they attach to their breaks, which do the job nicely. These checkpoints work like a lock-and-key system, as all receptors do. If the key fits, great. Once a key from another cell fits into the T-cell's checkpoint receptor, it switches it off, turning it into a lazy, good-for-nothing T-cell. Cancers use this built-in safety mechanism for their own benefit in a sneaky and nefarious way. The cancer cells turn on the checkpoints, relaying a message to the nearby T-cells to stand down, shutting the killer T-cell response off. Buggers.

Checkpoint *inhibitors* are drugs that block cancer cells' keys from binding to the T-cells checkpoint receptors, allowing the T-cells to start seeking and destroying all foreign invaders. One of the drawbacks of these inhibitors is that the immune response lacks specificity, often having negative consequences that look largely like autoimmune disease. But when they work, they can work very well. The checkpoint inhibitor class currently winning the race towards better cancer treatment inhibits the *programmed cell death protein 1* (PD-L1: a checkpoint receptor found on the T-cell) and *programmed death-ligand 1* (PD-1: one of the "keys" found on cancer cells). Since those names are long and sound kind of sinister, we just call them PD-1 and PD-L1. So today, the drugs with the most interest and research are the PD-1/PD-L1 inhibitors.

There are other classes of checkpoint inhibitors, such as the cytotoxic T lymphocyte antigen-4 (CTLA-4), which unfortunately doesn't have a bad-boy name, but is another mouthful. CTLA-4 is also a checkpoint used by cancer cells to turn off the T-cells, and the drugs that inhibit this break have also shown promise.

Adoptive Cell Therapies

Next up, we've got adoptive cell therapies, which aren't quite winning gold in this race for various reasons but are still super-impressive and have exciting potential. These use a process which makes good intuitive sense to most people. It's where a doctor harvests certain immune cells that can recognize a patient's tumour, multiplies them, then infuses them back into the patient's body. It's a treatment that holds a lot of promise for obvious reasons, but there are a lot of factors making it difficult to offer widely and effectively. There are currently two main treatments in this category: tumour-infiltrating lymphocytes (TILs) and chimeric antigen receptor T-cells (CAR-T). Bonus points to you for remembering any of these names.

Pathologists have long known that tumours usually contain TILs. These are Pac-Man cells that can recognize and destroy cancer cells, but the body often can't make enough of them to kill off the tumour. So, doctors have to artificially reproduce a whole bunch of them outside the body, and creating this volume is really flippin' hard, high-tech stuff. Also, this time and lab intensive process has to be done individually for each patient—no mass growing labs that can serve everyone. This makes it expensive as well. Another hit against this promising approach.

CAR-T cell therapy is next-level scientific innovation. Try your best to understand this one because you'll be happy if you do. Doctors first harvest a bunch of the patient's T-cells, then use an inactive virus to introduce genetic material into the T-cell DNA, prompting the T-cells to produce new receptors on their surface called *chimeric antigen receptors (CAR).* These special receptors are better able to find and bind cancer cells. In a lab, millions of these CAR-T cells are produced and then given to the patient, providing improved recognition of a given cancer. This has already shown to be effective in acute lymphoblastic leukemia and some non-Hodgkin lymphomas, and is showing promise in many other cancer types and other diseases.

Therapeutic Vaccines

The whole world is more conscious of vaccines today than ever before in human history. With the COVID-19 pandemic's international race to produce vaccines, we saw many of the world's pharmaceutical companies produce various types for this virus. If you followed these developments, you've had a quick lesson on inactivated viruses and modified RNA.

Amazingly, wonderfully, there are also vaccines for some cancers. These cancer vaccines are either autologous (which means they're made from the patient's own cells) or non-autologous (which means the vaccine uses a generic antigen common to the cancer).

The first FDA-approved cancer vaccine was for advanced (metastatic castration-resistant) prostate cancer. It is a customized vaccine made from the patient's own antigen presenting cells (autologous), namely dendritic cells, which are harvested from the patient's blood. In a lab, biochemists do a bunch of clever manipulations to these cells, then pop them back in the patient. Long story short, the dendritic cells are loaded with a prostate-specific antigen (protein), and once the dendritic cells are educated to go after the prostate protein, they are then infused into the patient.

Other FDA-approved vaccine therapies include dendritic cell vaccines, which are loaded with a patient's own cancer cell antigens. There are also oncolytic virus vaccines made from the pox virus and herpes simplex virus-1. In all these cancer vaccine approaches, cancer/tumour antigens are collected, cultured in a lab, activated by certain cytokines or viruses, then administered back into the patients. The hope is with all this clever immune stuff happening, it kills off the cancer. And on this cool work goes.

Non-specific Immune Stimulants

Finally, we've got non-specific immune stimulants. As the name suggests, these bad boys go everywhere, and they're not targeted. For example, certain cytokines like interferons and interleukins, like IFα, IL-2 and IL-6, from earlier in this book. They have been found to be somewhat successful and have been approved for use in "highly immunogenic cancers," including melanoma and renal cell carcinoma. Highly immunogenic means cancers which are particularly responsive to immune-directed treatments. The first positive study for the benefit of IF-α in treating melanoma was back in 1985.[89] The first study on IL-2 showing durable complete remissions in melanoma was in 1983, making this the first non-bug immunotherapy showing efficacy for human cancer patients. These continue to have some use today. Drawbacks to these cytokine immunotherapies include that they require prolonged use, are non-specific, and can cause significant side effects to the bone marrow and liver. Also, it now seems some of the newer, more targeted therapies can do a better job.

Another example of a non-specific immunotherapy has now been the standard treatment for bladder cancer since the mid-1980s. It uses Bacillus Calmette–Guérin (BCG), a live strain of the tuberculosis bug *Mycobacterium bovis*. With an intention and mechanism of action similar to that of Coley's, BCG has a much easier and better tolerated application. It's given via catheter directly into the bladder, so it doesn't affect anything else, and it triggers a local bladder immune response. The body thinks there's an infection there and goes into action to defeat it.

Probably the most commonly used non-specific immune stimulants today are what are called biological response modifiers (BMRs). These effectively promote the production of that good ol' fever-inducing cytokine IL-2. BMRs include thalidomide (yes, that thalidomide) and its derivates lenalidomide (Revlimid) and pomalidomide (Pomalyst).

You might remember the nightmares caused by thalidomide back in the day. It was prescribed for nausea and given to many pregnant women, but it damaged fetuses, caused awful congenital malformations and even deaths of newborns. However, its derivatives are now showing benefit for leukemias, where they increase the release of the fever-inducing, immune stimulating INF, IL-6, and TNF. A similar drug, Imiquimod, does the same thing on the body's surface, making it useful in skin cancers which are taken care of by the increased production of the INFs, ILs, and TNF. Cool how you know all of these cytokines now, and how the Pac-Man cells send these out to the immune system to take care of bad bugs or cells. You now also understand how all these immunotherapy treatments work.

With all four of these therapeutic approaches, we're occasionally seeing nice, robust responses. Yes, only in some cases and in certain cancers. But sometimes, when adequately able to stimulate that immune system, it's the answer. There is a long way to go, though. None of these treatments are yet effective in the majority of cases. The treatments need to be better tailored to each patient, and we need to do a better job of identifying what patients and cancers are most likely to respond to each treatment. We are now getting better at finding ideal patients by testing their cancer cells for the presence of PD-L1, microsatellite instability (high or not), mismatch repair gene, heavily mutated cells, and other factors that may make it more likely that immunotherapy will work.

My contention is that if we use such specific treatments affecting only one small part of the immune system, we will not win. That's like trying to change the entire score of a symphony by adjusting one note played by just one artist's instrument. There's only so much that such a small act can do. I submit that to truly change the sound, the conductor will have to adjust all or the majority of the musicians' music. And there are a couple of other treatments worth mentioning that induce a fever-like response to trigger the immune system into doing its beautiful business. They're not yet ready for primetime, but they have a long and interesting history worldwide.

Fever-range Whole-body Hyperthermia

One of these immunotherapy methods is fever-range whole-body hyperthermia (FR-WBHT), which has now been around since the 1950s. The German Society of Hyperthermia published the *Whole-Body Hyperthermia Guideline* in 2018, which gives the best current review of the scientific basis, evidence, indications, and applications.[90]

Rather than creating a true fever through the use of bacteria, viruses, and parasites that actually infect a patient, FR-WBHT heats the body from the outside using infrared-A light, creating an artificial fever. Although the initiation of the fever temperature is different, many of the same things happen once the body's core temperature is raised into the fever range of 38.5 to 40.5 Celsius. Many of the immune cells, cytokines, and systemic responses that occur throughout the body in real fever, also occur in FR-WBHT.

Here's how it goes down. Potential patients are thoroughly screened for pre-existing contraindications (or issues) including pre-existing heart problems, uncontrolled bleeding, swelling of the brain, very low hemoglobin or platelets, and a few others. But if all is good, the patient lies down on what looks like the lovechild of a hospital gurney and a sunbed. The doctor turns on the infrared-A light, then closely monitors the patient's temperature, blood pressure, heart, oxygen levels, and other vitals for the entire four- to six-hour, somewhat nightmarish, treatment. They also drip saline and dextrose through an IV line to keep the patient's blood pressure and sugars stable.

FR-WBHT raises the core body temperature into the human fever range of 38.5 to 40.5 degrees Celsius. This increases all of those Pac-Man cells including macrophages, natural killer cells. It increases the production of the cytokines TNF, IL-1, IL-2, IL-6.

As well as the bridging or antigen presenting cells like dendritic cells. Lastly, it increases the production of those smart yet killer T-cells.[91,92,93] The whole kit and kaboodle. This is much of the show you hope for from an actual fever from Coley's toxins or Klyuyeva's parasites. Without the risk of infection. No risk of it getting out of hand. But maybe some stuff is missing from the real thing.

I've overseen thousands of these FR-WBHT treatments during my career. Every patient makes it through, and everyone hates it. I mean, it feels like an actual fever. I know—I've suffered through it myself. It makes you hot, achy, and miserable. There's about a thirty-minute period where you want to crawl out of your skin, you're just so uncomfortable. Yet it's very safe, and everyone feels way better afterwards. When the fever breaks, it's like you've been through a profound detox, and a reset button has been pushed. You've sweated out a whole bunch, and you're left with this rosy sort of glow.

But cancer patients, in particular, don't care about that as much as their next scan results. And FR-WBHT can occasionally help produce some exceptional results. I've even seen complete remissions of advanced cancers. With the occasional wow clinical moments, it is consistently the case that most patients will experience significant improvements to their overall quality of life. This treatment also works outside of cancer therapy. There's evidence that people have had their severe, chronic depression lift for more than a year after going through this.[94] It's also been shown to effective in fibromyalgia.[95]

Of course, it may not be as ideal as creating a true endogenous fever, which is why it's called a hyperthermia treatment; the body's set point remains normal while the person is heated from the outside. This treatment gets close, but how to raise the core temperature *and* increase the set point? That would take us closer. But we still don't yet know how to artificially create a true fever safely. No one wants to repeat the risks of the Coley era.

FR-WBHT has benefits beyond the fever-like immune response and improvement to mood and physical condition. It enhances chemotherapy and radiotherapy when it used with those treatments. This is called *chemo-sensitizing* or *radio-sensitizing,*[96,97,98,99] meaning making chemotherapy and radiotherapy more effective. The same is proving true for partnering this treatment with immunotherapy drugs like our PD-1/PD-L1checkpoint inhibitor friends. Many patients also use FR-WBHT *after* going into remission to jump-start their immune system and help prevent a recurrence.

The widespread adoption of FR-WBHT is hampered by how difficult it is to administer. One doctor is with one patient for up to six hours. Above all else, there is an understandable lack of financial interest in such an onerous treatment. This explains the lack of research funding and interest, and thus large randomized trials.

Which, like most things in non-drug immunotherapy, are long overdue.[100] But more than five decades of use shows that this can be a safe and promising therapy, especially as part of a complete immunotherapy treatment approach.

Exciting, but Not Enough or Fast Enough

I have spent my entire professional life working one-on-one, face-to-face with human beings living with cancer. My patients all become experts in their disease, educating themselves on their options, doing all they can to stay alive as well and as long as possible. And they often ask me how we're doing with this whole cancer thing—if all the billions of dollars raised for cancer research every year are making a difference. Are we progressing? Are we "curing" cancer? Do we have any real answers? Of course, this is a complicated conversation, but one thing is clear to me: the progress, although real, has been frustratingly slow.

Let's be honest. We are still losing the fight on most cancers that have spread around the body. Here, we're losing badly. We have become better at treating cancer successfully when it can be found very early, cut out, and swept afterwards. There, we have become better in some cancers. But when someone's diagnosed with metastatic disease, and it's already spread to other parts of the body, there's been marginal differences in treatment success in the majority of cancers over the last century. Survival times have improved slightly here and there, but not much of a difference most of the time.

In my humble opinion, we are thankfully moving exponentially faster towards an answer to cancer, and that answer is in immunotherapy. I don't think we'll find the ultimate meaningful results in the DNA approach. We now know that the majority of metastatic cancers have a number of genetic mutations by the time they're found. Gene therapy will again need to hit a number of genes, rather than one at a time, to have a more meaningful impact. Chemotherapy and radiotherapy have been the mainstays for almost a century. They have held the fort. They have been the best answers for a long time, but with obvious limitations. As evidenced over the past few years, immunotherapy drugs are quickly replacing chemotherapy drugs. The future of immunotherapy is in discovering how to do this better. Because we know something important happens during an immune response, ultimately fever. We understand there are clinical benefits to recruiting the immune system to work for us. I suspect it won't be long before most chemo is replaced by more targeted immunotherapy. That's where we're headed.

It's tricky, though. It's clearly not as simple as, "Hey, go get a fever, and you'll be cured." No, just no. The body is too complex for that. And consider how individual those bodies are, with all the innumerable differences from one person to the next. That impacts a treatment's ability to produce an adequate immune response or not. Just think: Does the patient have adequate numbers of Pac-Man cells? Antigen presenting cells? T-cells? Are they sending out healthy cytokines? Are their receptors picking up the cytokine messages? Is their brain working? Do they have the calories needed to produce the response? Pharmacological research is complex, too. Chemical studies work by adjusting one variable at a time. Research might look at, say, PD-1 *or* PD-L1 *or* IL-1 *or* interferon or whatever. So, we have to ask, what does shifting each of these cells or cytokines do to the rest of the immune system's orchestra? And how do you possibly measure all that? You just can't.

I would like to see the pharmaceutical industry, and other smart laboratory researchers and clinicians, study all of those fever cytokines *together*. I mean, what happens if we go after PGE2, TNF, IL-1, IL-2, and IL-6 at the same time? My ideal fever therapy dream would be to intravenously administer a combination of all five of these biochemicals, and probably more, in a controlled manner. My hypothesis being that using lower dosages of each of these will prevent the unwanted side effects of each cytokine, but the synergy created with the combination will provide a robust fever response. A cocktail of these pyrogens would be able to induce a true, sustained, and controlled fever. As the dream continues, I would be able to carefully reverse that fever by introducing a cocktail of the endogenous cryogens, like arginine vasopressin, alpha-melanocyte-stimulating hormone, and whatever else is discovered, in order to bring the temperature back down. This is certainly in the realm of possibility right now, and I believe it's a solid goal for future research in industry and research centres alike. It's something I'd love to be part of.

However, we must remember that each of these cytokines is just one aspect of a brilliant, complex, multi-pronged, full-body orchestral response. I hope that one day, we can harness the immune system's ability to press fifty-odd buttons at once, triggering an orchestral response with trumpets playing here and drums banging there, all at the same time. Then, we'll really have something. For a better idea of what that might look—or rather, sound—like, let's talk next about our future with fever.

Chapter Ten: A Future with Fever

I have great respect for the past. If you don't know where you've come from, you don't know where you're going.

Maya Angelou, American author and civil rights activist, circa 1950

When you look inside a tumour, you'll see it's full of puss. What you can't see is that pussy stuff contains white blood cells called *tumour-infiltrating lymphocytes* (TILs).[101] TILs include all of those important immune cells we have previously discussed, the Pac-Man (innate), bridging (antigen presenting), and memory killer cells (cytotoxic T lymphocytes). Obviously, the immune system is doing its level best to try and attack those tumours. Science has long known that all of these cells hang out inside tumours, but not in all tumours equally. Some have more, some less. But here's the interesting thing: people whose tumours have the most TILs seem to end up living the longest.[102,103,104]

So, these magical TILs that correlate with the best survival rates are the immune system's soldiers that go into battle against the bad guys that are trying to infiltrate your defenses. TILs are critical in treating infections and cancer, so it's not surprising there's a direct relationship between how many TILs a person has and how long they survive against cancer. TILs are the cancer-killing and infection-fighting parts of the immune system, and you need a strong immune system to deal with cancer.

The presence of TILs in tumours confirms the fact that the immune system does indeed recognize cancer cells as foreign invaders, and tries its best to get rid of them. A well-functioning immune system equals better health, not just for fighting cancer but also many other diseases. So, we want to do whatever we can to improve our immune systems, right? The million-dollar question becomes how to get more, and more effective, good guy cells like these TILs. Not only that, but how do you also make the cancer cells look different enough that the immune system can recognize and get rid of them.

Despite the fact that we have known about these TILs since the early to mid 1900s, we still don't have an unequivocally proven, consistently effective, definitive treatment to increase and activate TILs. I know—it's disappointing for both of us. But we do have enough information today to point our research efforts to finding those definitive answers. Yeah, you guessed it, my contention is that we clearly should be looking towards fevers for answers.

A History of Afebrile Diathesis

There's a medical term called *afebrile diathesis. Afebrile* literally means *without fevers*, and *diathesis* means a tendency to suffer from a particular medical condition. So, afebrile diathesis, in everyday language, means a person has a personal medical history without any, or many, fevers through their life. Weird, right? People usually think that people who don't get fevers are healthy. They "never get sick." But let's take a closer look at this afebrile diathesis.

Time and time again, it's been observed and reported by physicians that patients diagnosed with cancer have had a striking lack of fevers throughout their lives. They note that their patients with an afebrile diathesis have a higher risk of cancer later in life.

As far back as 1854, the English ophthalmologist John Zachariah Lawrence wrote that patients with cancer had "a remarkable disease-free history."[105] But it was not until 1910 that the German physician K.L. Schmidt correlated a lack of fevers to an increased cancer risk in his study of 241 cancer patients, and actually coined the term *afebrile diathesis*.[106]

Two decades later, in 1934, another German doctor with the surname Engel compared 300 patients with cancer to 300 people without, finding a significantly increased risk of cancer in those people with an afebrile diathesis.[107,108] In 1977, Newhouse, Pearson and Fullerton published their study on 300 women with ovarian cancer and found significantly fewer incidences of mumps, measles, and rubella in those diagnosed with ovarian cancer compared to an age-matched control group.[109]

Lastly, in 1985, a Danish doctor called Tove Rønne linked "missing" childhood measles (which was common a few decades earlier, when the study participants were kids) with an increased risk for various cancers.[110] In his cohort of 353 people without childhood measles, 21 developed cancer. He compared them to a group of 230 patients with a positive history of measles. How many of them developed cancer? One. Just one. If you're a numbers kind of person, that means the hazard ratio was less than 0.001. Interesting, right?

I have certainly seen this afebrile diathesis in my own cancer clinic. Over the past quarter century, I have now had the privilege of working with thousands of people living with cancer. Being interested in immune and fever therapies, and this afebrile diathesis, I have asked thousands of my patients about their febrile history. The vast majority have reported that they haven't had fevers through their life. I haven't kept a formal record, but if I'd guess, this is true for over 80 percent of my queried patients. They typically say, "I never got sick much," or "I can't believe I was diagnosed with cancer doc, because I never get sick." This has now been documented repeatedly in the medical literature. Oncologists *keep saying* their patients haven't previously had fevers.

Of course, I'm not saying all you need to do to prevent cancer is get a fever. And I'm not suggesting that by getting fevers early on, you're guaranteed to live cancer-free. Cancer is complicated, and the human body is beautifully complicated. *But there is something to this fever thing.* As we've seen, despite all the advances, we are still losing the fight against cancer. We have to continue digging for answers. We certainly can't afford to ignore this critical data and empirical reports. Certainly, they're not definitive, but they are begging, pleading, and *screaming* for further research. Humanity and the scientific community at large need to continue to spend time and money figuring out exactly what happens during a fever, how it recruits our entire immune system, and how to turn this system on and off. We don't have all the answers yet, but we can't afford to ignore this any longer.

We Can't Afford to Wait

Right now, cancer is the leading cause of death worldwide according to the World Health Organization. In fact, the latest statistics suggest that 48 percent of men and 42 percent of women in the Western world will be diagnosed with cancer in their lifetime. That's one in two people! Look at the person sitting next to you. Statistically, one of you will get cancer. (Yes, I am the guy nobody wants to hang out with at a party.) And the rates are increasing.

Some people argue that this is because our technology has improved and we can now detect cancer sooner, but that's not entirely true. More people are dying from cancer now than ever before. We really are finding many cancers sooner, which should give us a better chance of doing something about it. But we're still not. More people are dying. And it's not just cancer that's on the up. More people have chronic infections, chronic diseases, and autoimmune conditions than ever before in our history.

We know there's an inextricable connection between cancer, as well as a myriad of other chronic health conditions, and the immune system. It's been proven again and again from all sorts of perspectives, in both animals and humans. Remember all those animal studies we discussed in chapter three? Researchers purposefully put bacteria and viruses into animals, then controlled their ability to fever. In those who are not allowed to build a fever, the infection is able to go unabated and takes their lives. But when animals can heat their bodies, their immune systems kick into action, and they overcome the disease.

Cancer is also more likely as people get older. What else happens when people age? Their immune systems become weaker. And think about COVID-19. As I write, there's still much more to learn on the subject, but it's already crystal clear that the elderly are most at risk, and that kids very rarely get it severely as adults. Why? At the simplest level, it's because younger people have more robust immune systems than ageing adults.

So, are you following along with me? Let's recap. TILs (that stuff in the puss) are an essential part of the immune response against anything deemed non-self, like a tumour. It has been repeatedly demonstrated that having more TILs in a tumour demonstrates a more robust immune attack against the cancer, creating a better chance of survival. And fevers increase TILs. Awesome. Next, fewer fevers throughout life increases the risk of cancer because the patient will have fewer TILs in their tumour, and therefore a greater chance of succumbing to cancer. Cancer is bad. So are other chronic diseases. We want strong immune systems, so we have to let our bodies fever.

Let the Army Practice

Imagine an army, buff and trim in all its battle gear, tanks at the ready, weapons meticulously cleaned, serviced, and ready for action. Then the general comes along and says, "Stand down, soldiers. Stay home, drink some beer, eat some crap, and have a smoke. We don't need ya." And more than that, the army isn't even allowed to train. No more practice. No drills. For *years*.

Then, a real enemy comes along. The general marches into the barracks and commands his troops into battle. Their time has come. Except, the soldiers have all got beer bellies now and iron lungs from all that smoking. They're not even sure where they left their gear, and when they find it, the weapons are rusted up. The troops run to gather in the quad, but they're coughing and wheezing before they get there. They're ill-prepared, to say the least. The enemy's going to walk all over them.

You know where I'm going with this, right? The army is your immune system. The enemy is cancer or something else ugly. If your army hasn't had the chance to practice, how will it take down the big, bad guys? You can't become the best fighter in the world without getting into a few scraps, then plenty more practice fights. This quote opens a chapter earlier in the book, but it's awesome, so I'll repeat it. "Fever is a mighty engine which Nature brings into the world for the conquest of her enemies." That comes from Thomas Sydenham, known as the father of English medicine, and he saw this was true back in 1650.

Maybe you're not into the fighting analogy. That's cool. Imagine your immune system is an orchestra. We've talked about how all the parts come together in harmony. But what if the trombone player never practices? What if none of the musicians have practiced? And, what if no one can remember how to tune the piano, none of the instruments have been maintained, and it's been so long since the conductor used his baton, he doesn't even know where it is anymore. Let's hear how harmonious *that* orchestra sounds.

My hypothesis is that in suppressing fevers repeatedly throughout our lives, we are muting our immune systems. I believe we should allow our immune systems to practice, get stronger, better, more effective and efficient. Otherwise, we are exchanging acute discomfort for chronic illness. We're swapping the noxious experience of fever for an immune system with no juice. And when the bad guys, like cancer, are so very bad, that is a problem.

Change Happens

Although we need more research, the information we have so far is beyond compelling. It tells us we need to change how we treat fevers. This change is not out of reach. In the past, we've changed our standards for all sorts of treatments. We talked about thalidomide in the last chapter. And let's talk about commonly prescribed antibiotics. There was a time when you'd go to the doctor feeling lousy with a congested chest, sore throat, phlegm coming out of everywhere, and the doctor would hand you some antibiotics to kill all the bad germs. Antibiotics, we believed, could handle so much stuff. They are amazing, but we now know that over 95 percent of respiratory tract infections (stuff with the upper throat, nose, sinuses, lungs, etc.) are *viral* infections—and antibiotics only kill bacteria. For decades and decades, doctors prescribed antibiotics that only kill bacteria for viral infections.

Of course, they thought it worked, and they were genuinely trying to help their patients. And who can blame them for trying whatever tools they had? I mean, imagine a patient desperately looking for help. They go see the doctor, who checks them out and says, "Oh, yeah, you're definitely sick. I want you to go home and rest." And the patient's like, "What? What do you mean *go home*? I'm sick. Give me something!" Even if the doctor suspects the problem is caused by a virus, such antivirals don't really exist, and who knows? Maybe it is bacterial. So, they prescribe antibiotics, and the patient merrily heads home, happy someone is doing something to help them.

Suddenly, bacteria like *Methicillin-resistant Staphylococcus aureus* (MRSA) show up, and, as the name implies, it doesn't respond to antibiotics. It is antibiotic-resistant, caused by the overuse of antibiotics. This became a major concern and the medical community acknowledged most respiratory tract infections were viral. So, doctors have now largely stopped prescribing antibiotics for them.

Tonsillectomies are another great example of positive change in medicine. When I was growing up, I had recurrent tonsillitis. That's where the tonsils at the back of the throat get all inflamed. You look inside your mouth and see these giant balls at the back of your throat, which are your tonsils. You get a sore throat and fever and have a hard time swallowing. It's not exactly dangerous, but it's a pain in the neck. Literally.

The standard treatment used to be surgery to whip those tonsils out. And it was *super* standard practice. I have two older sisters, and the three of us had our tonsils removed together, at the same time. The three of us were lined up in hospital beds eating Jello. I like to imagine the doctors had gone to our parents like, "Oh hey, Mr. and Mrs. Parmar. Good news! We can do you a special buy two, get one free offer. Let's do 'em all at once. Six tonsils, no waiting." My parents took the deal. Tonsils and adenoids, be gone.

So yeah, tonsillectomies—cutting those bad boys out—used to be common. And although I'm a little vintage, I'm not *that* old, so this wasn't that long ago. Now, though, the medical community understands tonsils are a major component of the immune system, protecting us as we breathe in bacteria and viruses. Tonsils are like our army barracks, housing the soldiers who check that what's coming in is okay. Occasionally, tonsillectomies do still happen when the kid is really suffering, maybe can't breathe right, and the parent doesn't want to put them through that any longer. But now that we know more, the standard practice of tonsillectomies has changed.

Doctors and Patients Together

It takes time for knowledge to accumulate, and doctors must do the best they can with what they have. Antibiotic use and tonsillectomies are great examples, though, of how we can improve worldwide standards of care once we know better.

Patients—you and me and everyone who ever sees a doctor—can help in this transition. Patients are so wise and knowledgeable these days. They do their own research, Google everything, and come to their doctors with their own information. In my world of oncology, my patients are *so* smart. As soon as they get their diagnosis, it's as if they're going to school to learn all they can.

Many patients tell me their other doctors hate how knowledgeable they are. I guess those docs just want to say, "This is the treatment. That's it." But my patients are asking questions, big time. They're asking about other treatments they read about. They're inquiring about test options. I love that. Yes, patients do have to be careful about getting reliable sources of information. I don't have to tell you there's a lot of weird stuff online. But when a source cites reliable medical information, it can be really useful to bring in that information and, along with your doctor, consider it for your situation. I'd love for you to do that with fever treatment, too. You can take an active role in your health and future immune system strength. You just need to know that sometimes, the best thing is nothing.

Hope for the Future

In 2002, a group at University College Medical School in England said, "New observations and discoveries have brought us to the point when we can move from the empirical to the rational approach. Many regarded as far-fetched the claims of Sir Almroth Wright that 'the physician of the future will be an immunizer', and he was unkindly nicknamed 'Sir Almost Right'. Yet in the field of cancer he may well be proved right. Certainly, our modern understanding of cancer and the immune phenomena associated with it gives us confidence to repeat Campbell De Morgan's assertion that we are encouraged to hope that a simple and highly effective cure may yet be found for the disease."[111] I have long maintained, and continue to, that the ultimate answer for cancer will be an immunological one.

The doctor they mention, Campbell De Morgan, lived in the 1800s. His thesis was that cancer started in one location, went to the lymph nodes, then spread elsewhere. Seems obvious now, but it wasn't back then. He also noted that cancer was uncommon in families affected by tuberculosis. See a theme here? De Morgan was convinced the answer for cancer lied somewhere in the immune system. He was unfailingly optimistic about the future of cancer, and I share that with him. With more research on how the immune system's surveillance and editing programs work, and how to get them pumping, we will find the treasures we seek.

We are in an arms race between us and everything else that lives on earth—bacteria, viruses, disease, and degeneration. That sounds bleak, but I can see a future where we are winning this battle. I imagine a world where people self-isolate when they're sick. Instead of taking NSAIDs and running around town, they stay home feeling lousy and feverish—and we all acknowledge that's a wonderful thing. I imagine people being praised for spreading less disease. I think about people letting their fevers ride, allowing their bodies to heal themselves, and, in the process, becoming stronger versions of themselves. Producing offspring with better immune systems, and over time we may see fewer chronic infections, less cancer, fewer autoimmune conditions, better mental health, and fewer people clogging up hospital emergency rooms, reducing the burden on healthcare systems.

I foresee a day when we are able to administer a specific intravenous cocktail of endogenous pyrogens (EPs) including IL-1, IL-2, IL-6, TNF, and PGE2 to induce a controlled fever response. I contend that using a cocktail of lower dose EPs will undoubtedly be more effective than using any one EP alone, providing a more natural, robust, and full-body fever response. By keeping the patient's core temperature in the fever range of 38.5-40.5 Celsius for as long as necessary to stimulate a profound fever-like response, the EP cocktail will prove safer and easier than using bacterial, viral, or parasitic infections. This may also be somewhat easier than using heating lamps to artificially raise the core temperature. Then, under careful observation and monitoring, endogenous cryogens (ECs) like anti-MSH and AVP could bring the fever down as needed.

It will take time to create this change, but I truly believe it is possible. We have all this information connecting illness and fever, so why are we trying to reinvent the wheel? Let's use the immune system as it was intended. Let's stop interfering with these intelligent processes our bodies evolved over hundreds of millions of years, and instead, let's employ fever to fight for us.

Conclusion

All truth passes through three stages. First, it is ridiculed. Second, it is violently opposed. Third, it is accepted as being self-evident.

Arthur Schopenhauer, German philosopher, circa 1800

Fever is a wise, ancient, evolutionarily conserved, powerful, and safe immune response that should be left alone to do its job in almost every case. Fever is something that we are all hard wired with to help ensure our survival, allowing our bodies to deal with harmful microbes and even cancer cells. In fact, as history has proven, fevers have been repeatedly documented to overcome advanced cancers.

Several treatments have been borne from our understanding of fever, and have proven effective against some cancers, including IL-2, IFN, and primed T-cell therapies, but an infinitely intelligent orchestra of fever will prove far more effective than any of these piece-meal treatments.

Further, by constantly suppressing fevers throughout our lives we weaken our immune systems, becoming more vulnerable to invaders. I believe that in allowing fevers to exercise their beautiful symphony we will be better immunologically protected against serious chronic diseases later in life. This last piece is the Hail Mary. As for the rest of it? No brainers, in my opinion. If we as a society continue interfering with fevers, there will continue to be a *tsunami* of illness.

We're already seeing this. We're living it right now. I mentioned this in the last chapter, but I want to repeat it here in case you skimmed through and missed it. (Hey, no judgement here!) Almost one in two adults (men a little more than women) in the Western world will be diagnosed with a cancer in their lifetime. Brutal, right? And the numbers aren't improving. Decade after decade, these percentages increase. More people are dying from cancer now than ever before.

Of course, this is due to myriad reasons including the ongoing pollution of our planet with innumerable carcinogens. Plus, more hours at work. More stress. Less sleep. Less exercise. Bad, bad food choices. Too much smoking. Too much booze. The list goes on. Many things are tough on our immune systems, not just the muting of our fever response. But this barrage of attacks makes it even more important to let our fever response thrive.

It's not just cancer that threatens us, either. More people are known to have chronic infections, diseases, and autoimmune conditions than at any other time in history. As I write, the COVID-19 pandemic has crippled our planet for almost two years, killing predominantly the elderly and the obese—again, those who don't have strong immune systems.

Despite all the world's advances in science and technology, we are not systemically getting better. Seven billion people on this planet will get fevers at some point of their life. And it's free.

With all those people and all these health issues, healthcare expenditures continue to rise worldwide. It's dangerous not only to our own bodies and wellbeing, but for our already overwhelmed medical systems and the economy.

Cancer is incredibly expensive to treat. Here in Canada, it's estimated that we spent about $4.4 billion of our tax base in 2017 on standard cancer treatment.[112] The cost for treatment is, of course, only one consideration. A 2021 Canadian publication estimated the many indirect costs of dealing with cancer. Annually per Canadian cancer patient, lost earnings averaged $8,200 for females and $3,200 for males; caregiver costs ranged from $15,786 to $20,414; household productivity losses were estimated to be up to $238,904 per household; friction costs incurred by employers were between $6,400 and $23,987; on a large scale, the societal productivity costs were estimated between $75 and $317 million.[113]

And that's cancer. COVID-19 has shown us what an entire world in medical crisis looks like, and it isn't pretty. Although the pandemic will thankfully come to an end, there are many other health challenges that will remain. By better understanding fever, we can make different choices about when to actively manage it and when it's better to rest, socially distance ourselves, and listen to our bodies.

Know Better, Do Better

We need to understand and help others realize the importance of temperature and how incredible our bodies are in regulating it—both in sickness and health. Notice that fever is essential throughout the animal kingdom, get curious about that, and realize we are part of that wonderful world. Know that interrupting fever does not just make sickness more tolerable but more long-lived and difficult to treat. Of course, this is a difficult subject because the history of fever and NSAIDs is not straightforward, and neither is the biochemistry involved in fever. Yet much of what we were raised to believe about fever is based on myths and misconceptions. With those dispelled, we know better and can do better. Despite the complexities, we can benefit from the body's natural immune system with immunotherapies, evolved from fever therapies to harness the body's innate wisdom. Remember that we can use the incredible power of the fever response to arm our immune systems and become stronger human beings.

I wrote this book as a public service announcement, and now I pass the torch to you to spread this essential message. We all have this incredible body mechanism that is a billion times better than any military on earth. It's constantly battling all sorts of offending agents. And it is always there for you—unless you shut it off. You have the power to engage that military by simply letting your fever ride. But realistically, you'll only do that when you don't *fear* fever. With the knowledge you now have, I hope you realize there's nothing to be scared of, and you understand the wonders of the immune system's fever response—how ubiquitous it is throughout the animal kingdom, how safe it is, how effective it is, and that it should be given the opportunity to help you when it arrives.

You can help your family, friends, colleagues, and loved ones see there's nothing to fear, so they too can become stronger, healthier, and better prepared for the future. I implore you to share these ideas, talk about what you've read, and discuss the challenges and opportunities in changing the standard of care for fever treatment.

This is already happening, hidden in research labs around the world, including in the USA at the MD Anderson Cancer Center in Texas, Duke University in North Carolina, and Roswell Park Comprehensive Cancer Center in New York. It's also going on in clinics and small hospitals like mine, where we're continuing the tradition of fever therapy to augment the immune system. Now, it's up to you to spread the word to your circles. Talk to the people you love. Have conversations with those involved in your health care. Push for deeper discussion, more research, and trust in our bodies. Together, our conversations can change our approach to fever management.

Beautiful and Essential

All those years ago, when I sat in that SFU lecture hall listening to Dr. Lawrence Dill talk about Darwinian Medicine and studying the book *Why We Get Sick*, I knew I was hearing something important. Not only did it spark an interest in fever and body temperature, but just generally how brilliant all living creatures are at protecting themselves from harm.

When you consider every part of our beautiful planet, the average temperature is 16 degrees Celsius, and it's been right around there for the entire time humans have existed. We have an average body temperature of 36 degrees. How the heck do we do that? Well, by now, you know how. We spend an absurd number of calories on maintaining our temperature. And when we go into crisis mode, we don't shut down and stop all that exhausting temperature management. No—we double down, spend even more energy, and raise our temperature.

This mechanism has survived and become critical over four hundred million years of refinement. Or on the other hand it was created in the image of God, and the big guy gave us this tool. Either way, our body's temperature management is so well established and works so well that we forget to notice it. But when we stop to consider, its sheer existence is mind-boggling. It simply would not exist if it weren't critical to our survival.

I'm happy to be sharing this important, age-old knowledge. I'm inspired by the incredible tireless efforts of the scientific and medical communities. I'm optimistic that this will help spark conversation and change. Bringing together ancient wisdom and new understanding. I am optimistic for the future of healthcare, and that we may all experience the ancient, beautiful, and beneficial effects of our fever response. We can all play a role in its guardianship, and provide this knowledge to our children, and they theirs. Trust the wisdom inherent in your body, arm your immune system, and share the incredible power of the fever response. Because when we honour our bodies, we can be sick less, get better faster, and live healthier lives.

Acknowledgements

I would like to thank my teachers.

My family and friends. Thank you for making daily life rich, and the motivation to be better.

To all my academic teachers, most recently my writing coach Liz Green.

Lastly, to my long-time tennis coach Fu, thanks for teaching me that tennis is a perfect metaphor for life.

References

Introduction

[1] Kluger MJ. *Fever: Its Biology, Evolution, and Function.* Princeton University Press; 1979.

Chapter One

[2] Starks PT, Blackie CA, Seeley TD. Fever in honeybee colonies. Naturwissenschaften. 2000. 87:229-231.

[3] Simone-Finstrom M, Foo B, Tarpy DR, Starks PT. Impact of Food Availability, Pathogen Exposure, and Genetic Diversity on Thermoregulation in Honey Bees (Apis mellifera). *J Insect Behav.* 2014;27(4):527-539. doi: 10.1007/s10905-014-9447-3

[4] Kluger MJ. *Fever: Its Biology, Evolution, and Function.* Princeton University Press; 1979.

[5] Kluger MJ. *Fever: Its Biology, Evolution, and Function.* Princeton University Press; 1979.

[6] O'Grady NP, Barie PS, Bartlett JG, et al. Guidelines for evaluation of new fever in critically ill adult patients: 2008 update from the American College of Critical Care Medicine and the Infectious Diseases Society of America [published correction appears in Crit Care Med. 2008 Jun;36(6):1992]. *Crit Care Med.* 2008;36(4):1330-1349. doi:10.1097/CCM.0b013e318169eda9

[7] Kluger MJ. *Fever: Its Biology, Evolution, and Function.* Princeton University Press; 1979.

8 Popson MS, Dimri M, Borger J. Biochemistry, Heat and Calories. In: *StatPearls*. Treasure Island (FL): StatPearls Publishing; June 26, 2021.

9 Altman PL, Dittmer DS. Vol III Biology Data Book, 2nd Ed. *Fed. Amer. Soc. Exp. Biol.* 1974.

10 Giesbrecht GG. Cold stress, near drowning and accidental hypothermia: a review. *Aviat Space Environ Med.* 2000;71(7):733-752.

11 Walter EJ, Hanna-Jumma S, Carraretto M, Forni L. The pathophysiological basis and consequences of fever. *Crit Care.* 2016;20(1):200. Published 2016 Jul 14. doi:10.1186/s13054-016-1375-5

12 Wright WF, Mackowiak PA. Origin, Evolution and Clinical Application of the Thermometer. *Am J Med Sci.* 2016;351(5):526-534. doi:10.1016/j.amjms.2015.11.019

13 Payne JF. *Thomas Sydenham*. London: T Fisher Unwin; 1900.

14 Wright WF, Mackowiak PA. Origin, Evolution and Clinical Application of the Thermometer. *Am J Med Sci.* 2016;351(5):526-534. doi:10.1016/j.amjms.2015.11.019

15 Taylor. 1942.

16 Wright WF, Mackowiak PA. Origin, Evolution and Clinical Application of the Thermometer. *Am J Med Sci.* 2016;351(5):526-534. doi:10.1016/j.amjms.2015.11.019

17 Taylor FS. The origin of the thermometer. *Annals of Science.* 1942. 5:129-156.

18 Wright WF, Mackowiak PA. Origin, Evolution and Clinical Application of the Thermometer. *Am J Med Sci.* 2016;351(5):526-534. doi:10.1016/j.amjms.2015.11.019

19 Taylor FS. The origin of the thermometer. *Annals of Science.* 1942. 5:129-156.

[20] Pasteur L. Memoire sur les corpuscles organizes qui existent en suspension dans l'atmosphere. Examen de la doctrine des generations spontanees. *Ann Sci Nat.* 1861;16:5-98.

[21] Snell ES, Atkins E. The mechanisms of fever. *The Biological Basis of Medicine.* 1968:397-419.

Chapter Two

[22] Kluger MJ. Fever: role of pyrogens and cryogens. *Physiol Rev.* 1991;71(1):93-127. doi:10.1152/physrev.1991.71.1.93

[23] Cooper KE, Cranston WI, Snell ES. Temperature regulation during fever in man. *Clin Sci.* 1964. 27:345-356.

[24] Lwoff A. Death and transfiguration of a problem. *Bacteriol Rev.* 1969;33(3):390-403. doi:10.1128/br.33.3.390-403.1969

Chapter Three

[25] Edleston RS. [No title]. *Entomologist.* 1864;2:150.

[26] Kettlewell HBD. *The Evolution of Melanism. The Study of a Recurring Necessity.* Clarendon Press; 1973.

[27] Rice SA. *Encyclopedia of Evolution.* Facts on File; 2007:308.

[28] Kluger MJ. Fever: role of pyrogens and cryogens. *Physiol Rev.* 1991;71(1):93-127. doi:10.1152/physrev.1991.71.1.93

[29] Mackowiak PA. Physiological rationale for suppression of fever. *Clin Infect Dis.* 2000;31 Suppl 5:S185-S189. doi:10.1086/317511

[30] Atkins E, Bodel P. Fever. *N Engl J Med.* 1972;286(1):27-34. doi:10.1056/NEJM197201062860109

[31] Kluger MJ, Ringler DH, Anver MR. Fever and survival. *Science.* 1975;188(4184):166-168.

[32] Vaughn LK, Veale WL, Cooper KE. Antipyresis: its effect on mortality rate of bacterially infected rabbits. *Brain Res Bull.* 1980;5(1):69-73. doi:10.1016/0361-9230(80)90285-3

[33] Husseini RH, Sweet C, Collie MH, Smith H. Elevation of nasal viral levels by suppression of fever in ferrets infected with influenza viruses of differing virulence. *J Infect Dis*. 1982;145(4):520-524. doi:10.1093/infdis/145.4.520

[34] Mackowiak PA. Physiological rationale for suppression of fever. *Clin Infect Dis*. 2000;31 Suppl 5:S185-S189. doi:10.1086/317511

Chapter Four

[35] Stitt JT. Prostaglandin E as the neural mediator of the febrile response. *Yale J Biol Med*. 1986;59(2):137-149.

[36] Kluger MJ. Fever: role of pyrogens and cryogens. *Physiol Rev*. 1991;71(1):93-127. doi:10.1152/physrev.1991.71.1.93

[37] Plaisance KI, Mackowiak PA. Antipyretic therapy: physiologic rationale, diagnostic implications, and clinical consequences. *Arch Intern Med*. 2000;160(4):449-456. doi:10.1001/archinte.160.4.449

[38] Norn S, Permin H, Kruse PR, Kruse E. From willow bark to acetylsalicylic acid. Fra pilebark til acetylsalicylsyre. *Dan Medicinhist Arbog*. 2009;37:79-98.

[39] Mackowiak PA. Physiological rationale for suppression of fever. *Clin Infect Dis*. 2000;31 Suppl 5:S185-S189. doi:10.1086/317511

[40] Agrawal S, Khazaeni B. Acetaminophen Toxicity. [Updated 2021 Jul 18]. In: StatPearls [Internet]. Treasure Island (FL): StatPearls Publishing; 2021 Jan-. Available from: https://www.ncbi.nlm.nih.gov/books/NBK441917/

[41] Drake TM, Fairfield CJ, Pius R, et al. Non-steroidal anti-inflammatory drug use and outcomes of COVID-19 in the ISARIC Clinical Characterisation Protocol UK cohort: a matched, prospective cohort study. *Lancet Rheumatol*. 2021;3(7):e498-e506. doi:10.1016/S2665-9913(21)00104-1

42 Abu Esba LC, Alqahtani RA, Thomas A, Shamas N, Alswaidan L, Mardawi G. Ibuprofen and NSAID Use in COVID-19 Infected Patients Is Not Associated with Worse Outcomes: A Prospective Cohort Study. *Infect Dis Ther.* 2021;10(1):253-268. doi:10.1007/s40121-020-00363-w

43 Acetaminophen vs. NSAIDs during COVID-19 pandemic. Therapeutics Initiative. March 18, 2020. Accessed September 16, 2021. https://www.ti.ubc.ca/2020/03/18/acetaminophen-vs-nsaids-during-covid-19-pandemic/

Chapter Five

44 Doran TF, De Angelis C, Baumgardner RA, Mellits ED. Acetaminophen: more harm than good for chickenpox? *J Pediatr.* 1989;114(6):1045-1048. doi:10.1016/s0022-3476(89)80461-5

45 Stanley ED, Jackson GG, Panusarn C, Rubenis M, Dirda V. Increased virus shedding with aspirin treatment of rhinovirus infection. *JAMA*. 1975;231(12):1248-1251.

46 Graham NM, Burrell CJ, Douglas RM, Debelle P, Davies L. Adverse effects of aspirin, acetaminophen, and ibuprofen on immune function, viral shedding, and clinical status in rhinovirus-infected volunteers. *J Infect Dis.* 1990;162(6):1277-1282. doi:10.1093/infdis/162.6.1277

47 Bryant RE, Hood AF, Hood CE, Koenig MG. Factors affecting mortality of gram-negative rod bacteremia. *Arch Intern Med*. 1971;127(1):120-128.

48 Mackowiak PA, Browne RH, Southern PM Jr, Smith JW. Polymicrobial sepsis: an analysis of 184 cases using log linear models. *Am J Med Sci*. 1980;280(2):73-80. doi:10.1097/00000441-198009000-00002

49 Weinstein MP, Iannini PB, Stratton CW, Eickhoff TC. Spontaneous bacterial peritonitis. A review of 28 cases with emphasis on improved survival and factors

influencing prognosis. *Am J Med*. 1978;64(4):592-598. doi:10.1016/0002-9343(78)90578-8

[50] Gozzoli V, Schöttker P, Suter PM, Ricou B. Is it worth treating fever in intensive care unit patients? Preliminary results from a randomized trial of the effect of external cooling. *Arch Intern Med*. 2001;161(1):121-123. doi:10.1001/archinte.161.1.121

[51] Ray JJ, Schulman CI. Fever: suppress or let it ride?. *J Thorac Dis*. 2015;7(12):E633-E636. doi:10.3978/j.issn.2072-1439.2015.12.28

[52] Dallimore J, Ebmeier S, Thayabaran D, et al. Effect of active temperature management on mortality in intensive care unit patients. *Crit Care Resusc*. 2018;20(2):150-163.

[53] Mackowiak PA. Physiological rationale for suppression of fever. *Clin Infect Dis*. 2000;31 Suppl 5:S185-S189. doi:10.1086/317511

Chapter Six

[54] Pathogenesis of Fever. *Clinical Manual of Fever in Children*. 2009;47-61. doi:10.1007/978-3-540-78598-9_3

[55] Veale and Cooper. 1975.

[56] Page LA. High body temperature of pigeons and sparrows as a factor in their resistance to an agent oof the Psittacosis group. *Bull Wildl Dis Assoc*. 1965;1(4):49-53.

[57] Pathogenesis of Fever. *Clinical Manual of Fever in Children*. 2009;47-61. doi:10.1007/978-3-540-78598-9_3

[58] Kluger MJ. Fever: role of pyrogens and cryogens. *Physiol Rev*. 1991;71(1):93-127. doi:10.1152/physrev.1991.71.1.93

Chapter Seven

[59] Hippocrates, Jones WHS. *Hippocrates Volume IV: Nature of Man Regimen in Health. Humours. Aphorisms. Regimen 1–3. Dreams*. Loeb Classical Library; 1931.

[60] Bryant RE, Hood AF, Hood CE, Koenig MG. Factors affecting mortality of gram-negative rod bacteremia. *Arch Intern Med*. 1971;127(1):120-128.

[61] Mackowiak PA, Browne RH, Southern PM Jr, Smith JW. Polymicrobial sepsis: an analysis of 184 cases using log linear models. *Am J Med Sci*. 1980;280(2):73-80. doi:10.1097/00000441-198009000-00002

[62] Weinstein MP, Iannini PB, Stratton CW, Eickhoff TC. Spontaneous bacterial peritonitis. A review of 28 cases with emphasis on improved survival and factors influencing prognosis. *Am J Med*. 1978;64(4):592-598. doi:10.1016/0002-9343(78)90578-8

[63] Young P, Saxena M, Bellomo R, et al. Acetaminophen for Fever in Critically Ill Patients with Suspected Infection. *N Engl J Med*. 2015;373(23):2215-2224. doi:10.1056/NEJMoa1508375

[64] Young PJ, Bailey MJ, Bass F, et al. Randomised evaluation of active control of temperature versus ordinary temperature management (REACTOR) trial. *Intensive Care Med*. 2019;45(10):1382-1391. doi:10.1007/s00134-019-05729-4

[65] Mackowiak PA. Physiological rationale for suppression of fever. *Clin Infect Dis*. 2000;31 Suppl 5:S185-S189. doi:10.1086/317511

[66] Mackowiak PA. Physiological rationale for suppression of fever. *Clin Infect Dis*. 2000;31 Suppl 5:S185-S189. doi:10.1086/317511

[67] Kluger MJ. *Fever: Its Biology, Evolution, and Function*. Princeton University Press; 1979.

[68] Mackowiak PA. Physiological rationale for suppression of fever. *Clin Infect Dis*. 2000;31 Suppl 5:S185-S189. doi:10.1086/317511

[69] Young PJ, Bellomo R, Bernard GR, et al. Fever control in critically ill adults. An individual patient data meta-

analysis of randomised controlled trials. *Intensive Care Med.* 2019;45(4):468-476. doi:10.1007/s00134-019-05553w

Chapter Eight

[70] Coley WB. The treatment of malignant tumors by repeated inoculations of erysipelas. With a report of ten original cases. 1893. *Clin Orthop Relat Res.* 1991;(262):3-11.

[71] Hobohm HU. *Healing Heat: An Essay on Cancer Fever Therapy.* BoD-Books on Demand; 2016.

[72] MacAdam DH. *The Reinvention of Coley's Toxins.* Donald H. MacAdam; 2018.

[73] Coley WB. II. Contribution to the Knowledge of Sarcoma. *Ann Surg.* 1891;14(3):199-220. doi:10.1097/00000658-189112000-00015

[74] Coley WB. The treatment of malignant tumors by repeated inoculations of erysipelas. With a report of ten original cases. 1893. *Clin Orthop Relat Res.* 1991;(262):3-11.

[75] Busch, W. Aus der sitzung der medicinischen section vom 13 November 1867. *Berl Klin Wochenschr.* 1868;5:137.

[76] Fehleisen F. Uber die Zuchtung der Erysipelkokken auf kunstlichem Nahrboden und die Ubertragbarkeit auf den Menschen. *Dtsch Med Wochenschau.* 1882;8:553.

[77] Coley WB. The treatment of malignant tumors by repeated inoculations of erysipelas. With a report of ten original cases. 1893. *Clin Orthop Relat Res.* 1991;(262):3-11.

[78] Coley WB. The treatment of malignant tumors by repeated inoculations of erysipelas. With a report of ten original cases. 1893. *Clin Orthop Relat Res.* 1991;(262):3-11.

[79] Kluger MJ. Fever: role of pyrogens and cryogens. *Physiol Rev.* 1991;71(1):93-127. doi:10.1152/physrev.1991.71.1.93

[80] Starnes CO. Coley's toxins in perspective. *Nature.* 1992;357(6373):11-12. doi:10.1038/357011a0

[81] Ramírez-Toloza G, Ferreira A. *Trypanosoma cruzi* Evades the Complement System as an Efficient Strategy to Survive in the Mammalian Host: The Specific Roles of Host/Parasite Molecules and *Trypanosoma cruzi* Calreticulin. *Front Microbiol.* 2017;8:1667. Published 2017 Sep 1. doi:10.3389/fmicb.2017.01667

[82] Klyuyeva NG, Roskin GL. *Biotherapy of Malignant Tumours*. Pergamon Press; 1963.

[83] Tsay CJ. Julius Wagner-Jauregg and the legacy of malarial therapy for the treatment of general paresis of the insane. *Yale J Biol Med*. 2013;86(2):245-254.

[84] Challenor S, Tucker D. SARS-CoV-2-induced remission of Hodgkin lymphoma. *Br J Haematol*. 2021;192(3):415. doi:10.1111/bjh.17116

Chapter Nine

[85] Association of the British Pharmaceutical Industry. *Oncology Mission Report, US East Coast, November 2000.* London: Association of the British Pharmaceutical Industry, 2001.

[86] Shankaran V, Ikeda H, Bruce AT, et al. IFNgamma and lymphocytes prevent primary tumour development and shape tumour immunogenicity. *Nature*. 2001;410(6832):1107-1111. doi:10.1038/35074122

[87] Corthay A. Does the immune system naturally protect against cancer?. *Front Immunol.* 2014;5:197. Published 2014 May 12. doi:10.3389/fimmu.2014.00197

[88] Finn OJ. Immuno-oncology: understanding the function and dysfunction of the immune system in cancer. *Ann Oncol.* 2012;23 Suppl 8(Suppl 8):viii6-viii9. doi:10.1093/annonc/mds256

[89] Kirkwood JM, Ernstoff M. Melanoma: therapeutic options with recombinant interferons. *Semin Oncol.* 1985;12(4 Suppl 5):7-12.

[90] Parmar G, Kazcor T. *Textbook of naturopathic oncology: a desktop guide of integrative cancer care.* Medicatrix Holdings Ltd; 2020;8:459-477.

[91] Evans SS, Repasky EA, Fisher DT. Fever and the thermal regulation of immunity: the immune system feels the heat. *Nat Rev Immunol.* 2015;15(6):335-349. doi:10.1038/nri3843

[92] Kobayashi Y, Ito Y, Ostapenko VV, et al. Fever-range whole-body heat treatment stimulates antigen-specific T-cell responses in humans. *Immunol Lett.* 2014;162(1 Pt A):256-261. doi:10.1016/j.imlet.2014.09.014

[93] Romeyke T, Stummer H. Multi-modal pain therapy of fibromyalgia syndrome with integration of systemic whole-body hyperthermia – effects on pain intensity and mental state: A non-randomised controlled study. *J Musculoskel Pain* 2014;4:341-55.

[94] Janssen CW, Lowry CA, Mehl MR, et al. Whole-Body Hyperthermia for the Treatment of Major Depressive Disorder: A Randomized Clinical Trial [published correction appears in JAMA Psychiatry. 2016 Aug 1;73(8):878]. *JAMA Psychiatry.* 2016;73(8):789-795. doi:10.1001/jamapsychiatry.2016.1031

[95] Romeyke T, Stummer H. Multi-modal pain therapy of fibromyalgia syndrome with integration of systemic whole-body hyperthermia – effects on pain intensity and mental state: A non-randomised controlled study. *J Musculoskel Pain* 2014;4:341-55.

[96] Sakaguchi Y, Makino M, Kaneko T, et al. Therapeutic efficacy of long duration-low temperature whole body hyperthermia when combined with tumor necrosis factor and carboplatin in rats. *Cancer Res.* 1994;54(8):2223-2227.

[97] Viglianti B, Stauffer P, Repasky E, Jones E, Vujaskovic Z, Dewhirst M. *Holland-Frei Cancer Medicine 8*. Waun Ki Hong et al., ed. Vol 8. 8th ed. PMPH-USA; 2010.

[98] Vaupel P. Tumor microenvironmental physiology and its implications for radiation oncology. *Seminars in Radiation Oncology*. Vol 14. Elsevier; 2004:198-206.

[99] Masunaga S, Nagata K, Suzuki M, Kashino G, Kinashi Y, Ono K. Inhibition of repair of radiation-induced damage by mild temperature hyperthermia, referring to the effect on quiescent cell populations. *Radiat Med*. 2007;25(8):417-425. doi:10.1007/s11604-007-0160-4

[100] Ohguri T, Imada H, Korogi Y, Narisada H. Clinical results of systemic chemotherapy combined with regional hyperthermia. *Nippon Haipasamia Gakkai-Shi*. 2007;23(2):49-61.

Chapter Ten

[101] Black MM, Opler SR, Speer FD. Structural representations of tumor-host relationships in gastric carcinoma. *Surg Gynecol Obstet*. 1956;102(5):599-603.

[102] Galon J, Angell HK, Bedognetti D, Marincola FM. The continuum of cancer immunosurveillance: prognostic, predictive, and mechanistic signatures. *Immunity*. 2013;39(1):11-26. doi:10.1016/j.immuni.2013.07.008

[103] Galon J. Prognostic markers of the immune system-immune infiltration into the tumour. *Eur. J. Cancer*. 2012;48: 7–8.

[104] Mei Z, Liu Y, Liu C, et al. Tumour-infiltrating inflammation and prognosis in colorectal cancer: systematic review and meta-analysis. *Br J Cancer*. 2014;110(6):1595-1605. doi:10.1038/bjc.2014.46

[105] Laurence JZ. *The Diagnosis of Surgical Cancer (Liston Prize Essay for 1854)*. London: John Churchill; 1855.

[106] Schmidt KL. Krebs und Infekcionskrankheiten. *Med Klinik Wschr.* 1910;43:1690-1693.

[107] Engel P. Ober den Infektionsindex dee Krebskranken. *Wien Klin Wschr.* 1934;47:1.

[108] Engel P. Ober den Einfluß des Alters auf den Infektionsindex der Krebskranken. *Wien Klin Wschr.* 935;48:ll2.

[109] Newhouse ML, Pearson RM, Fullerton JM, Boesen EA, Shannon HS. A case control study of carcinoma of the ovary. *Br J Prev Soc Med.* 1977;31(3):148-153. doi:10.1136/jech.31.3.148

[110] Rønne T. Measles virus infection without rash in childhood is related to disease in adult life. *Lancet.* 1985;1(8419):1-5. doi:10.1016/s0140-6736(85)90961-4

[111] Grange JM, Stanford JL, Stanford CA. Campbell De Morgan's 'Observations on cancer', and their relevance today. *J R Soc Med.* 2002;95(6):296-299. doi:10.1258/jrsm.95.6.296

Conclusion

[112] De Oliveira C, Pataky R, Bremner KE, et al. Estimating the Cost of Cancer Care in British Columbia and Ontario: A Canadian Inter-Provincial Comparison. Estimation du coût des soins contre le cancer en Colombie-Britannique et en Ontario: une comparaison interprovinciale au Canada. *Healthc Policy.* 2017;12(3):95-108.

[113] Iragorri N, de Oliveira C, Fitzgerald N, Essue B. The Indirect Cost Burden of Cancer Care in Canada: A Systematic Literature Review. *Appl Health Econ Health Policy.* 2021;19(3):325-341. doi:10.1007/s40258-020-00619-z

CPSIA information can be obtained
at www.ICGtesting.com
Printed in the USA
BVHW040206040322
630520BV00005B/17